MEMORIZING PHARMACOLOGY

A Relaxed Approach, Second Edition

Tony Guerra, M.HCI., Pharm.D.

Memorizing Pharmacology: A Relaxed Approach, Second Edition

Tony Guerra, M.HCI., Pharm.D.
ISBN: 978-1-957259-00-0

To Mindy,
Brielle, Rianne, and Teagan

AUTHOR'S NOTE

WHAT'S IN THIS UPDATE?

As I wrote *Memorizing Pharmacology: A Relaxed Approach*, I wanted to make it a lot easier for students to learn the Top 200 drugs and over 50,000 students enjoyed that book. In this expanded edition, where you can memorize even more pharmacology faster, I now have mnemonics for over 300 medications as a response to the various licensing exams adding so many more medications. The goal of this book is the same though, give students who are strapped for time a way to quickly learn pharmacology.

In addition to more medications and more mnemonics, you'll find over 150 questions with answers and rationales. I also go through my process of tackling dosage calculations, and making it easier to remember just where to start with each question and helping you calm that math anxiety.

So, let's get on with this updated edition, and helping you make it through pharmacology class and beyond.

THE STORY OF PHARMACOLOGY CLASS

As an instructor, I didn't appreciate how tough it was to be a working parent and pharmacology student until I had my triplet daughters. When the girls originally came home, they had trouble coordinating the suck, swallow, breathe that goes with feeding from a bottle, well, three bottles. We fed them for 90 minutes and they slept for

90 minutes – round the clock. They got older, but the crushing emotional and physical exhaustion has continued. Most of my students have jobs and families. I wanted a way for them to study pharmacology while attending to these types of responsibilities.

Tonight, as I lay quietly in bed next to my daughter who will not sleep otherwise, **I recited in my head, from memory, the 300 drugs, generic name, brand name and drug classification, in this book, in order.** Previously during these times, thoughts of "What do I have to do for tomorrow?" ran through my head. Instead, I could relax, stay unhurriedly by my daughter, and remain a committed parent. With this book's techniques, I could study pharmacology in the dark – eyes closed. I knew I was on to something. This could help my overworked students.

After she fell asleep, I got up and starting writing this introduction, but before I could congratulate myself, my other daughter came downstairs insisting that she will never sleep in her bed again. So, here I am, on my couch, half-watching *Better Call Saul*, comforting another daughter between coughing fits, and typing out this introduction, knowing I might see the sunrise before I get to sleep.

Earlier this fall a student emailed me, offering to pay me to read and record his "Top 300 Drugs" list. I was too busy mid-semester, but I did want to create a road map for him and other students that shared his need. Each fall and spring, many health professional students try to learn the "Top 300 Drugs," but get little help in memorization techniques.

This book *will* help, regardless of which Top 100, 200, or 300 Drugs your professor assigns.

TOP 300 DRUGS – A HISTORY

What does Top 300 Drugs mean? At one time, there was a website that listed The Top 300 Drugs in the United States by 1) Number of prescriptions written and 2) Ranked by money spent on each drug. This created two different lists, but their value was clear. **Well-prepared students remember the most frequently prescribed drugs.** The 80/20 rule, or Pareto's principle, predicts that 20% of the medications will represent 80% of those prescribed.

Brutal rote memorization, however, is a poor strategy for managing information overload. Memorizing a brand name, generic name, medication class, therapeutic use, and one adverse effect for 300 drugs represents one-thousand pieces of information. Each new item adds 300 disparate memorization points. Students often ask why they should memorize drugs if they can Google them or look them up in a *Davis Drug Guide for Nurses*. The answer: a properly sorted and memorized list of 300 drugs provides a framework on which to build your preparation for pharmacology class, the board exams, and clinical practice. But, how did *I* memorize so many drugs? Follow this thought experiment.

Imagine, instead of playing the part of student, you are the instructor. The class has 300 students and there are exactly 300 seats in the classroom. How do you remember all of their names? How do you know who is absent when you see empty chairs? You could ask the students to sit alphabetically by first name or by last name, but this is college, not grade school. A more organic approach would take time to understand why groups formed as they did.

Students sit in the same seats weekly. As you talk and get to know them, you find out what brings them together. They may have the same undergraduate major, hometown, dorm, previous class, and so forth. There are the front row groups that always asks questions or back row group that asks no questions. Groups come from the same hospital floor or work on a semester project. If someone's absent, you know what group he or she are missing from.

As you learn the drugs in this book, you'll see similar groupings. For example, you'll see a gastrointestinal drugs group, an SSRI antidepressant section, benzodiazepines together, and angiotensin-converting enzyme inhibitors next to the angiotensin-II receptor blockers. When you bring medicines back from memory, you'll remember if one is missing.

This book provides that specific framework to memorize the most important drugs in a logical order. A good analogy is that learning to drive a car requires essentially the same foundational instruction. However, once you learn, you can drive anywhere (or anything) you want. After you learn *this* list, you can insert and delete drugs.

We have a problem, however, because pharmacology instructors and students speak different languages. This causes instructors to get student comments like "He can't teach," "I didn't learn anything in his class," and "C's get degrees, I guess." Professors who cannot connect to students frustrate those who want to learn. I am especially empathetic to parents and students with full-time jobs and international students trying to pick up English *and* the language of pharmacology. I am a parent of three daughters and English is not my first language. Let me show you this disconnect between a student's and a teacher's memorization metaphors.

Pharmacology breaks down to "pharmaco" or "drug" and "logy" which is "study of" with a connecting "o" to make "study of drugs." There is another concept called *pharmacokinetics*. "Pharmaco" means "drug" and "kinetics" means movement, like a kinesiology major is someone who studies – "logy" – body movement – "kinesio."

When, as a pharmacology instructor, I look at the word *pharmacokinetics*, I think of four major principles: *absorption*, *distribution*, *metabolism*, and *excretion*. I remember the A-D-M-E mnemonic, pronounced: "add-me." I remember each principle as matching a certain organ or tissue.

- Absorption happens in the *small intestine's* villi.
- Distribution occurs via the *blood.*
- Metabolism happens in the *liver.*
- Excretion occurs through the *kidneys.*

With my anatomy and physiology background, I memorized these facts through a metaphor of connected tunnels. A drug travels from the mouth to the small intestine to be *absorbed* and then through blood vessels to be *distributed* to the liver where it's *metabolized*. Eventually it goes through the kidneys to be *excreted*, further passing through the ureters, into the bladder, and the urethra. That picture is clear and complete in my brain.

I used to assume that my students, some of whom took anatomy and physiology, learned it the same way. That wasn't true. When asked to create a writing prompt of how they memorized the same idea, my students used a different set of metaphors.

One equated *absorption* with soaking up material in a classroom, *distributing* knowledge to short- and long-term memory, *metabolizing* the information down into manageable topics, and *excretion* to eliminating extraneous pieces of information.

Another student condensed a semester's worth of developmental psychology into a sentence. She associated the increased surface area of her pregnant belly with the intestine's *absorption*; *distribution* with the bloodline that she imparts to her child; changes in her life to accommodate the child, including possibly future drinking after pregnancy, to remember the *metabolism* in the liver; and *excretion* as the expulsion of the child from her home after high school.

After reading that story, can you tell me what *pharmacology* and *pharmacokinetics* mean? Whose story did you use, the instructor's or the student's? I don't think one is better than the other is, but it can be helpful to have a more complete understanding through two points of view.

THE CURSE OF KNOWLEDGE

This divide between expert and novice has a name – "The Curse of Knowledge." When you have been an expert at something, but you just can't explain it to someone, it might be because you understand the whole process and they are just learning step-by-step. The same is true in pharm.

Whatever pharmacology text you are using has an author trying to tell the same story from a different expert point of view to novice audiences. I've found pharmacology books specifically titled for allied health, athletic training, audiologists, dental hygienists, EMS providers, health professions, massage therapists, medical assistants, medical office workers, nurses, paramedics, pharmacists, pharmacy technicians, physical therapists, physicians, rehabilitation professionals, respiratory care therapists, surgical technologists, veterinary technicians and veterinarians. I stopped counting at twenty. Even as someone writes a textbook, the base of knowledge expands and changes. The better approach starts with a general primer like this, a very small amount of information, 300 drugs in this case, and expands from it. Then a student can take what he or she specifically needs from discipline-specific pharmacology textbooks.

I have read many of those discipline-specific books and taught in many disciplines, but you get the point – **pharmacology is an ever-expanding subject too big to distill; it's best learned by acquiring a base and building up from there.** I would recommend that you find out how your fellow students learn, but in a big lecture hall, you often don't talk to classmates. This book picks up not only the shortcuts those students use to help them get a better grade in pharm, but also their methods.

TAKING PHARMACOLOGY TWICE, SORT OF.

Most of the above-mentioned pharmacology textbooks have the same basic format. The early chapters cover the interactions of the drugs with the body, *pharmacodynamics*, and the body on the drug, *pharmacokinetics*, along with introducing some basic vocabulary. The author divides chapters by pathophysiologic condition and medications follow, e.g., gastrointestinal medicines, then cardiac medicines, and so forth.

However, many sections rely on understanding material from a future section. The instructor has a full overview of all the knowledge, but the student doesn't. Soon, the instructor is talking over the student's head. Here is an example: What medications treat an ulcer and why?

A student can memorize the three medications, **omeprazole (Prilosec), amoxicillin (Amoxil),** and **clarithromycin (Biaxin)** that comprise an ulcer treatment regimen. However, to move up Bloom's taxonomy from knowledge (memorizing "what") to comprehension (understanding "why") requires significant additional information.

- **Omeprazole (Prilosec)**, a proton pump inhibitor, reduces stomach acid and gains an advantage over **calcium carbonate (Tums)** and **famotidine (Zantac)** because of its extended half-life, a measure of the time it takes for a drug in the body to reduce by half.

- **Amoxicillin (Amoxil)** kills the causative agent in most ulcers, *Helicobacter pylori*, a helicopter- shaped bacterium that's sensitive to penicillin antibiotics.

- **Clarithromycin (Biaxin)** reduces the incidence of resistance that can happen with a single broad-spectrum antibiotic like **amoxicillin (Amoxil).**

Instructors teach **omeprazole (Prilosec)** in the earlier gastrointestinal section. Weeks later, students learn how **amoxicillin (Amoxil)** and **clarithromycin (Biaxin)** work in the antimicrobial section of the course. This second major point is critical – **To learn pharmacology requires that a student has already taken pharmacology.** This seems ridiculous, but let's use an apt metaphor, a trip to another country.

CREATING A PRIMER

Imagine you will start college in the fall and have decided to take a four-credit Spanish class. You could hope the teacher slows down to whatever speed you need, or you could study ahead of time. Let's pretend you decide to travel to the Peruvian mountains. (That happens to be where my dad is from.) Although some people speak English, you ask them to speak to you in Spanish so they can help you learn Spanish for your class. Your smartphone doesn't get any signal in the Andes Mountains, so you use pen and paper to write your notes in a small journal, picking up words along the way. At first, you point to objects but, gradually, you can start making sentences. You make notes of words that are especially tricky. For example, the Spanish word embarazada *looks like* the English word embarrassed, but it *means* pregnant. If you make this mistake, your brain will remember the story of that mistake, and you won't make it again. You compare notes with other students and share stories each night. In the end, you have a primer, an introductory book in Spanish that will put you far ahead of your class as you enter college.

The word "primer" has different meanings in various contexts. In auto painting and cosmetics, a primer allows for better adhesion for a secondary product's application. A primer is also a basic language-reading textbook. You can combine these definitions to create a useful analogy. **A pharmacology primer can provide a home base for students to expand a basic framework of vocabulary before they use PowerPoints (sentences) and textbooks (full paragraphs).**

This book is your journal. In the same way you take medical terminology before you take anatomy and physiology, you want to master some of the terms before you start pharm class. The following seven chapters include conversations with students about creating meaning from words in the foreign language of pharmacology. I will talk through how and why I have grouped them as I did. Once you have completed the book, the Comprehensive Drug List should look like conversational and readily pronounceable English.

MEDICATION RECONCILIATION (MED REC)

While this book's focus is to prepare students, I believe it can help patients and caregivers provide accurate medication histories and records – as students of their own conditions. Medication reconciliation or "med rec" is the process of assembling a correct list of patient's medications under what might be some stressful circumstances. When an ambulance comes, you might not remember to take everything with you. Memorizing medications in a logical order ensures the list will always be with you and you can immediately tell EMS responders what the patient is on.

FINAL NOTE

If you pass your pharmacology class, feel free to email me:

tonythepharmacist@gmail.com

I want to share in your victory and I'm always looking for better ways to teach pharm. If you see a student struggling with the language of pharmacology who doesn't have this book or a patient who wants to better understand his or her many prescriptions, please do take the time to recommend it to them.

There was a pharmacology class that I got a standing ovation, just like in the 1972 movie *The Paper Chase*. I hope what you get out of this book is worth your standing up.

Table of Contents

Contents

Contents

Contents

Contents

Contents

Contents

INTRODUCTION

GENERIC NAMES VS. BRAND NAMES

From experience, instructors immediately know which names represent *generic* and *brand* drugs. In an academic text, generic names go first in lower case letters followed by a capitalized brand name in parenthesis, e.g., **amphotericin B (Fungizone)**. In conversation or other writing, students must have this distinction memorized.

Some licensing exams only use generic names. This is understandable; only one generic name exists for each medication. There is one "**acetaminophen**," but the brand **Tylenol** is associated with many products. This *does not* mean a student should *not learn* brand names. A dangerous confusion between generic and brand names is that of **Pepto-Bismol** or **Pepto** for short. Let me tell you a story.

On a web page I saw a parent post that she gave her 8-year-old child a teaspoonful of **Pepto**, was that okay? **Pepto-Bismol** is the brand name for the liquid product **bismuth subsalicylate**. That salicylate is similar to **aspirin**, which is **acetylsalicylic acid** and can cause a terrible condition called **Reye's syndrome** in children. What she meant to give her child was **Children's Pepto**, which contains **calcium carbonate**, the active ingredient in **Tums**. As a parent, I understand what happens in the middle of the night. Your child is suffering and the medication instructions are in tiny 4-point font. It's tough to make the right call.

1

The point is that most brand names will have two to three syllables (**Pepto**). Most generic names have four or more: **calcium carbonate** and **bismuth subsalicylate**. Why is this important?

You want to start developing simple *heuristics,* or rules of thumb, to make it easier to learn the medicines. For example, generic names have stems like the "-cillin" in penicillin class antibiotics; brand names do not. Getting meaning from a brand or generic requires a different rule of thumb. If you don't know if the drug name you are looking at is generic or brand, you are at a terrible disadvantage.

THREE TYPES OF DRUG NAMES

1) The chemical name: First, there is the most complex name, the International Union of Pure and Applied Chemistry (IUPAC) standard name, which makes perfect sense to a chemist who might want to draw the molecule. For example, **Ibuprofen's** chemical name is:

(RS)-2-(4-(2-methylpropyl)phenyl) propanoic acid

Chemists may simplify the chemical name. In this example, the chemical name becomes the common name, Iso-butyl-propanoic-phenolic acid (I bu pro phen), which can be shortened even further to ibuprofen, the generic name.

2) The generic name: With only four syllables, the transformation to **ibuprofen** is an improvement over the chemical name. Patients, however, prefer two to three syllable names. Just as kids cut down computer to "puter" or banana to "nana," patients prefer short names for ease of pronunciation.

If you don't know where to put an emphasis on a generic four syllable drug name, it's usually the penultimate, or second to last, so it would be pronounced **i bu PRO fen**.

You want to make sure to put the right *emphasis* on the right *syllable* or you'll lose credibility. If your patient pushes the call button when you walk *into* the room, you might be mispronouncing some meds.

3) The brand or trade name: Two of the brand names for **ibuprofen** are **Advil** and **Motrin**. Both have two easy-to-pronounce syllables, but don't resemble **ibuprofen** as the brand name because they include *plosives* to make powerful memorable stops in the word. A strong word sounds like strong medicine.

Say each of the following letters and see if you can feel it in your tongue or nose.

Tongue blade occlusion: *t or d*

Tongue body occlusion: *k or g*

Lip occlusion: *b or p*

Nasal stops: *m or n*

Motrin has an "m," a nasal stop; a "t," a tongue blade occlusion; and an "n," another nasal stop. This forces the person saying the word to stop their breath three times, slowing the pronunciation and keeping it on the tongue and / or nose longer, making it sound very strong.

BRAND NAME RULE OF THUMB: CAN INDICATE FUNCTION

The **brand name's** two to three syllables will sometimes hint at the *function* of a drug, i.e., **Lopressor** <u>low</u>ers blood <u>pres</u>sure

The **brand name** is similar to a two- to three-syllable nickname that *hints* at the drug's function, but by law, may not make a claim. Brand names are very much like nicknames such as Betsy or Jack. A non-native English speaker would have no idea that Betsy comes from Elizabeth or Jack comes from Jonathan. Betsy takes the "b-e-t" from Elizabeth and Jack takes the "J" from Jonathan.

You might see brand names do the same, such as the use of "val" in the brand name **Valtrex** (an antiviral), which comes from a part of the generic **<u>val</u>acyclovir** or the "p," "a," and "x" in the brand name **<u>Pax</u>il** (an antidepressant), which come from the generic name <u>pax</u>etine.

GENERIC NAME RULE OF THUMB: CAN INDICATE CLASS

Lopressor's four syllable generic name, **metoprolol (Toprol, Toprol XL)**, has an –olol suffix, which is a **stem** from a credible source.

I know of two stem lists. One is from the **United States Adopted Names Council** on the American Medical Association's website and another is the **World Health Organization's** (WHO) Stem Book. They created stems so when people use generic names, they will know that the drugs with similar stems are probably similar in their actions. This is where the problems start.

Students, recognizing similarities in the endings or beginnings of drug names, start to make up their own rules.

In this book, you will learn which stems are credible and verifiable and which are not. Knowing both will make you much better at spotting them. Most YouTube videos and Quizlet notecards have errors that let you know the author's research is faulty or nonexistent. I am not picking on students; many licensed health professionals give advice and charge money online to view their videos, and some of that advice is dead wrong. However, when used correctly, these prefixes, suffixes, and infixes can be invaluable.

Some of the references, online videos, and online pre-made note cards provide lists deriving stems incorrectly. For example, the nine endings -azole, -en, -ide, -in, -ine, -one, -pam, -sone, and -zine are *not* stems; these are only groups of letters that happen to be at the end of many medication names. Using a group of letters instead of an established stem might lead to a drug classification error.

PREFIXES, SUFFIXES, AND INFIXES

In this book, I will use the terms prefix, suffix, and infix. Generic drug names are invented words and do not always conform to the rules of English. The United States Adopted Names Council properly calls each prefix and suffix that has meaning (e.g., cef- represents cephalosporins or –cillin represents penicillins) a stem.

In the case of penicillin, -cillin is the stem and peni- is a prefix that differentiates peni*cillin* from other penicillin antibiotics such as amoxi*cillin* or ampi*cillin*, etc.

An infix is inside the word to make the classification more specific. The proper stem for a quinolone antibiotic is –oxacin, but cipro*floxacin* has the infix –*fl*- to classify it further as a *fluoro*quinolone, one that contains a fluorine atom.

Stems work as a heuristic, or something that allows us to accelerate our recognition of a class of medications. If there is a list of ten medications that all end in –olol, we can more easily know these medications are beta-blockers.

The stem –adol indicates a drug like **tram<u>adol</u> (Ultram)**, is an analgesic (a medication for pain), comprised of an opiate (which means from the opium poppy, but is more generally a term for many narcotics). This has properties as both an agonist (a chemical that stimulates a receptor) and an antagonist (a chemical that blocks or antagonizes a receptor), which is unusual. Usually a chemical is an agonist or antagonist, not both.

The stem -afil in **silden<u>afil</u> (Viagra)** and **tadal<u>afil</u> (Cialis)** represents the phosphodiesterase type-5 (PDE5) inhibitors and indicates that these medications block (inhibit) an enzyme (phosphodiesterase). The inhibition of this enzyme results in stopping the breakdown of a chemical in the corpus cavernosum. This effect helps patients who have erectile dysfunction.

The stem –amivir in **oselt<u>amivir</u> (Tamiflu)** and **zan<u>amivir</u> (Relenza)** is a subclass of the stem –vir that represents the neuraminidase (enzyme) antagonist (inhibitor) group. Neuraminidase is an enzyme critical for influenza virus replication. If the medication in given in a certain time frame, usually within the first 48 hours after symptom onset, it blocks the enzymes necessary for influenza viruses to successfully replicate.

The stem "–azepam" represents antianxiety agents in the benzodiazepine class that are similar to **di<u>azepam</u> (Valium)**. Besides anxiety, patients use these medications as a sedative-hypnotic.

That's a lot of information to get from a few letters.

PRONUNCIATION AND ORGANIC CHEMISTRY WORD PARTS

Pronouncing generic names is often like pronouncing foreign language last names like mine. My last name "Guerra" has a part that's unpronounceable in regular English because there is no double or rolled "r" sound in English. Drug names might use the same letters you know in the Roman alphabet. However, we pronounce them differently because the sounds that form them come from organic chemists and biochemists.

Note: Below I have italicized the part of the generic name to which the organic molecule corresponds. These are *not* classification stems like –cillin or –azepam, but references to certain chemicals or groups of them.

These words indicate the number of carbon atoms in an attached molecule made up of only carbon and hydrogen atoms:

Methyl – *Methyl*phenidate	*METH-ill*
Ethyl – Fentan*yl*	*ETH-ill*
Propyl – Meto*prol*ol	*PROP-ill*
Butyl – Alb*ut*erol	*BYOUT-ill*

Levo and dextro mean left and right respectively:

Levo - *Levo*thyroxine	*LEE-vo*
Dextro - *Dex*methylphenidate	*DEX-trow*

These words mean there is a specific element in each molecule:

Thio (sulfur) – Hydrochloro*thio*azide	*THIGH-oh*
Chloro (chlorine) – Hydro*chloro*thiazide	*KLOR-oh*
Hydro (hydrogen) – *Hydro*codone	*HIGH-droe*

7

Fluoro (fluorine) – Cipro*flo*xacin   *FLOR-oh*

These words are branches that attach to the central molecule:

Acetyl – Levetir*acet*am	*Uh-SEAT-ill*
Alcohol – Tramad*ol*	*AL-kuh-haul*
Amide – Loper*amide*	*UH-myde*
Amine – Diphenhydr*amine*	*UH-mean*
Disulfide – *Disulf*iram	*DIE-sulf-eyed*
Furan – *Fur*osemide	*FYOOR-an*
Guanidine – Cimet*idine*	*GWAN-eh-dean*
Hydroxide – Magnesium *Hydroxide*	*HI-drox-eyed*
Imidazole – Omepr*azole*	*im-id-AZ-ole*
Ketone – Spironolac*tone*	*KEY-tone*
Phenol – Acetamino*phen*	*FEN-ole*
Sulfa – *Sulfa*methoxazole	*SULL-fuh*

Some chemists name drugs:

- By what they do for the patient, also called the therapeutic class: Anti-depressant
- By their chemical structure: Tricyclic antidepressants (TCAs) (three rings in the compound)
- By the receptor they affect: Beta-blockers
- By the neurotransmitter they affect: Selective serotonin reuptake inhibitor (SSRI)

You will become familiar with these classifications as we progress through the book. That's another big reason you want to be around other people when discussing the medications. You will pick up the pronunciation as you make mistakes or listen to others make mistakes. There is no shame in this; it's a part of learning. You cannot exactly pick up pronunciation from looking at brand and generic names. However, if you pay attention to drug names, you will find clues for building strong mnemonics.

Homophones

In grade school, you may have learned the word "homophone." Homophones are words that sound the same, but that we spell differently. Some examples include the words "there" and "their," "two" and "too," and "hear" and "here." To remember which meaning is associated with the word, your teacher may have told you to look inside the word for a clue.

In the word "their" you find "heir," such as the person who will inherit something. Then you can associate that the word "their" has to do with the possessive form of a group of people versus "there" which means "in that place."

In the word "two," you can turn the "w" sideways to make a 3, spelling "t3o" to remember that two has to do with a number. Also, "too" has two o's, and you can remember that it has too many o's.

In the word "hear" you find the word "ear," which reminds you this word means to listen, versus "here" which means "in this place."

Those clues are mnemonic devices, something to help your memory. Mnemonics also work in the memorization of drugs.

Note: The word mnemonic comes from the name Mnemosyne, the goddess of memory in Greek mythology.

Mnemonics in pharmacology

The brand name **Prilosec**, a proton pump inhibitor for reducing stomach acid, contains "Pr" which can be short for "proton" (H^+), the ion associated with something acidic.

Prilosec contains "l-o" which can be short for "low" as in the opposite of high. **Prilosec** contains "sec" which can be short for "secretion."

Prilosec's mechanism of action (MOA) is to inhibit proton pumps and reduce the acid in a person's stomach. By looking at the name of the drug, we can see that "proton" "low" "secretion" means a reduction in protons, helping us remember the meaning of the word.

However, if you only remembered the generic name, **omeprazole**, and forgot what the stem –prazole meant or what the drug was for, you would be in trouble. Brand names serve as a back-up plan.

When developing my mnemonics, I did not call anyone at any brand name drug companies. I just looked at each drug name and used my experience as a teacher of pathophys, pharmacology, and organic and biochemistry, and made up something that seems to make sense, but that, more importantly, will help students remember the drug's drug class and / or function. The FDA does not allow a drug company to name a drug after its intended use, but there are hints in many drug names that you can definitely see.

3 BY 5 NOTECARDS

Many students prefer to use notecards rather than just relying on a book. I think you can get everything you need from this book alone, but I know that 3 by 5 notecards you *make* are much better than any you can *buy*. A book from Harvard University Press titled *Make It Stick: The Science of Successful Learning*, by Peter Brown, goes into why generative (making things) learning is so important.

Notecards are portable. You can sort them and challenge others to sort them like UNO or playing cards. To help you along, I have created a specific order that makes sense out of these 200 cards so you know *how* to sort them. The "how to sort them" aspect is the next level of learning beyond memorizing the purpose of drugs or their generic and brand names.

Drugs next to each other are related and those within a group are in a larger family based on physiologic system. As you go through the book, you will see connections between the drug before and after the one you are studying.

You will also see what *types* of connections are available in addition to those you know already. We will take small steps, but I know you will be impressed when you can name every single drug's brand name, generic name, and class from memory.

Here is what a notecard might look like:

3x5 card front:
famo<u>tidine</u>

3x5 card back:
Class: H_2 blockers have the stem "-tidine." Looks like "to dine," which can be associated with GERD.

The brand name **Pepcid** has the "pep" from peptic, which means digestion, and the "cid" from acid.

COMPREHENSIVE DRUG LIST DISCUSSION

I didn't make this three-page list to intimidate you. It's just that if you spread out 200 3 x 5 notecards, 10 down and 20 across, it makes an area 4 feet by 8 feet. This list helps you see the whole forest – connections between drugs and stems unapparent in a stack of cards.

Start by memorizing the seven pathophysiologic classes in this book in order as G-M-RINCE, as Grand Mothers RINCE kids' hair (except it's the French r-i-n-c-e instead of the English r-i-n-s-e) to set up the broadest framework. These seven pathophysiologic classes will be the steel reinforcing bars that, when surrounded by concrete, will provide the foundation for your memorizing the gastrointestinal (G), musculoskeletal (M), respiratory (R), immune (I), neuro (N), cardio (C), and endocrine (E) systems' medications.

This G-M-RINCE order places drug classes from easiest to hardest to learn. To make it easier to memorize the whole thing, I had to create some simple rules – a computer programmer might call these algorithms. In each section, these are the two major rules:

1. Each of the seven sections has over-the-counter medications presented first and then prescription medications after. I present all OTC gastrointestinal products before all RX products, so the drugs consumers can physically interact with at the pharmacy come first.

2. I alphabetized drugs in the same class unless there is a pharmacologic reason to consider them out of alphabetical order.

For example, **diphenhydramine**, a 1st-generation antihistamine that starts with "d," would go before **cetirizine**, a 2nd-generation antihistamine that starts with "c." The generational move from 1st to 2nd overrides the alphabetical order. However, **cetirizine** and **loratadine** are both 2nd generation antihistamines so those *are* in alphabetical order. Therefore, the order becomes **diphenhydramine**, **cetirizine**, **loratadine** – one first-generation and two second-generation antihistamines.

This is how our brains work – ever consolidating and organizing until meaning emerges from a compact, somewhat fractured list. The ultimate goal is to consolidate all seven chapters in the comprehensive drug list. You shouldn't need 300 notecards to memorize 300 drugs; you should only need 12 – one for each group.

CHAPTER 1
GASTROINTESTINAL

I. PEPTIC ULCER DISEASE

Clinicians diagnose peptic ulcer disease (PUD) when an ulceration of the peptic or digestive tract occurs. Acid is an aggressive factor in the stomach that, if reduced, allows an ulcer to heal. In this chapter we'll focus on antacids, histamine$_2$ receptor antagonists (also known as H$_2$ blockers), and proton pump inhibitors. Note: antibiotics eradicate *Helicobacter pylori*, the organism responsible for the ulcers, but we will tackle those in chapter 4.

ANTACIDS

Antacids, or literally, anti-acids, can contain the elements **calcium** and **magnesium** to raise the stomach's pH. The *pH scale* is like a one-foot long ruler with 14 lines instead of 12. A "0" sits left for the most acidic compounds and a "14" sits right for the most basic or alkaline ones. 7, which is in the middle, is neutral. Stomach acid has a pH of 2; milk is 6; neutral is 7; and blood is 7.35. Why give dairy milk, which is slightly acidic, to calm an acidic stomach? Because 6 is more basic (alkaline) than 2.

Besides acting as an antacid, **calcium carbonate (Tums)** can supplement calcium in a diet and **magnesium hydroxide (Milk of Magnesia)** works as a laxative. Unfortunately, both antacids can **chelate** (bind with) antibiotics like **doxycycline (Doryx)** and **ciprofloxacin (Cipro).**

Calcium carbonate (Tums, Children's Pepto)
CAL-see-um CAR-bow-nate (TUMS)

> Students associate the brand name Tums with the word tummy to remember it's an antacid. **Calcium carbonate (Children's Pepto)** and **bismuth subsalicylate (Adult Pepto-Bismol)** have different ingredients and should not be interchanged.

Magnesium Hydroxide (Milk of Magnesia)
mag-KNEES-e-um high-DROCKS-ide (MILK mag-KNEE-shuh)

> **Milk of Magnesia** looks like dairy milk, which can work similarly to an antacid in calming an acidic stomach. Put together the "milky texture" and the diarrhea of lactose intolerance to remember its laxative effect.

HISTAMINE2 RECEPTOR ANTAGONISTS (H2RAS)

The term H_2 blocker (more formally, H_2 receptor antagonist) stands for histamine receptor type two (H_2) blocker. Histamine2 causes the formation of acid, so blocking its receptors reduces the production of acid. You will notice **cimetidine (Tagamet)**, **famotidine (Pepcid, Zantac),** and **nizatidine (Axid)** both end in "tidine." Related drugs often have related stems in their names.

When someone says, "I need an antihistamine," they are generally looking for relief from allergic symptoms like sneezing, runny nose, watery eyes, etc. Those allergy antihistamines affect histamine one (H_1) receptors. We will cover those in the respiratory chapter. The following H-2 blockers have the "-tidine" stem.

Cimetidine (Tagamet)
sigh–MEH–tih–dean (TAG-uh-met)

> **Tagamet** takes some letters from antagonist, as these
> are H-2 antagonists. Cimetidine has many drug
> interactions and is often a poor therapeutic choice.

Famotidine (Pepcid, Zantac)
Fa–MOE–tih–dean (PEP-sid, ZAN-Tak)

> **Pepcid** contains "pep" from "peptic" and "pepsin"
> that relates to digestion, and "cid" from "acid." One
> student mentioned Pepsi, the soda, has a pH of 2.4,
> which is very acidic. She said it always gave her
> heartburn, so that's how she remembered **Pepcid**.
> Also, in soda pop, the "p-o-p" and **Pepcid's** "p-e-p"
> are very similar. Note, brand **Zantac** changed the
> active ingredient from ranitidine to famotidine once
> rantidine was pulled from the shelves.

Nizatidine (Axid)
Nigh–ZAH-tih–dean (AK-sid)

> **Axid** is the word acid with a letter "x" replacing the
> letter "c" indicating what the drug reduces.

PROTON PUMP INHIBITORS (PPIs)

Proton pump inhibitors (PPIs) block a pump that introduces
protons (which are acidic) into the stomach, thus making it
less acidic. Prescribers combine PPIs with antibiotics for
ulcer triple therapy to kill *H. pylori*.

While **esomeprazole (Nexium)** and **omeprazole (Prilosec)**
have the same ending "prazole," notice the only thing that
separates **omeprazole** and **esomeprazole** is an "es." Many
drugs have chemical structures that have mirror images
called enantiomers. Instead of calling them right- and left-

handed, we call them "R" and "S" from the Latin words *rectus* (right) and *sinister* (left).

In this case, the "S" form is more active biologically. Putting an "s" in front of omeprazole would make "someprazole," which would be pronounced "some-prazole." Instead, the prefix "es" allows for a separation between the "S" sound and the compound name, as a chemist would pronounce it.

Dexlansoprazole (Dexilant)
decks-lan-SOAP-rah-zole (DECK-sih-lant)

> **Dexilant** stands for *right-handed excellent* because the right-handed enantiomer lasts longer than its racemic lansoprazole counterpart does. Dexlansoprazole is the (R)(+) enantiomer of lansoprazole and could be considered superior.

Esomeprazole (Nexium)
es-oh-MEP-rah-zole (NECKS-see-um)

> Again, the "prazole" ending means PPI and the "e-s" means "S" for sinister or left-handed active molecule. The manufacturer released **Nexium** after **Prilosec** as the "next" PPI drug.

Omeprazole (Prilosec)
oh-MEP-rah-zole (PRY-low-sec)

> We remember **Prilosec** by the "Pr" for hydrogen protons (protons, or hydrogen ions, are what make an acid acidic), the "lo" for low, and the "sec" for secretion of those protons. Or, the "o" in Prilosec looks like a zero, and **Pril-"O"-sec** provides zero heartburn.

Lansoprazole (Prevacid)
lan-SOAP-rah-zole (PREH-vuh-cid)

Prevacid will "<u>prev</u>ent <u>acid</u>."

Pantoprazole (Protonix)
pan-TOE-prah-zole (PRO-taw-nicks)

> **Protonix** "<u>ni</u>xes <u>pro</u>tons" or gets rid of protons. Pantoprazole, like esomeprazole and rabeprazole, comes in an IV form.

Rabeprazole (AcipHex)
ruh-BEH-prah-zole (AS-uh-feks)

> **AcipHex** combines "a-c-i" from <u>aci</u>d, "pH" (little p capital H) from the <u>pH</u> scale, and "ex" meaning to get rid of

II. Diarrhea, IBS, Constipation, and Emesis

Diarrhea can lead to dehydration and sometimes we need to intervene and use over-the-counter medications like **bismuth subsalicylate (Pepto-Bismol)** or **loperamide (Imodium)**. **Diphenoxylate with atropine** represents the increase in the aggressiveness of treatment from OTC to prescription.

Bismuth's "**subsalicylate**" is similar to aspirin (acetyl**salicy**lic acid), and is dangerous to young children. **Bismuth subsalicylate (Pepto Bismol)** is not appropriate for children because of the risk of **Reye's syndrome**, a condition involving brain and liver damage that can occur in children with chicken pox or influenza who take **salicylates**.

Irritable bowel syndrome, IBS, can include cramping, constipation and/or or diarrhea, but we see **dicyclomine**

(Bentyl) and Hyoscyamine) for these which can also work for diarrhea.

Opioids like **morphine (Kadian)** decrease gastrointestinal tract motility, causing constipation. Calcium channel blockers like **verapamil (Calan)** block calcium from getting to the bowel's smooth muscle. Prescribers frequently give a stool softener like **docusate sodium (Colace)** and a stimulant laxative for constipation caused by these medications, or due to other causes.

Emesis or vomiting is an effective natural body response to ingested toxins. However, with cancer chemotherapy, we want to prevent chemotherapy-induced nausea and vomiting (CINV) with drugs like **ondansetron (Zofran)**.

Manufacturers specifically formulate these meds because nausea patients may vomit oral meds. For example, **ondansetron (Zofran)** comes as an orally disintegrating tablet (ODT) that patients take without water, and **promethazine (Phenergan)** as a rectal suppository.

Antidiarrheals

Bismuth Subsalicylate (Pepto-Bismol)
BIZ-muth sub-sal-IS-uh-late (pep-TOE BIZ-mol)

> The "b" in **bismuth subsalicylate** reminds students of the black tongue and black stool that some patients experience as side effects. (Note: This discoloration is harmless.) **Pepto** looks like peptic, which has to do with digestion.

Loperamide (Imodium)
Low-PER-uh-mide (eh-MOE-dee-um)

The "lo" for s<u>lo</u>w and "per" for <u>per</u>istalsis is how a student remembered **loperamide's** function. **Imodium** is like the word "immobile" in that it slows down the bowel.

Diphenoxylate / <u>atro</u>pine (Lomotil)
die-fen-AWK-suh-late / AH-truh-peen (LOH-muh-til or Luh-MOAT-ul)

The brand name **Lomotil** spells out "<u>low</u> <u>moti</u>lity" for slowing down diarrhea. The **atropine** is there to prevent someone from crushing the **diphenoxylate** and injecting it illicitly.

IRRITABLE BOWEL SYNDROME (IBS)

Dicyclomine (Bentyl)
Die-SIGH-klu-mean (BEN-till)

Dicyclomine is an anticholinergic which relaxes smooth muscles reducing GI spasms. However, anticholinergics can cause dry eyes, mouth, and even constipation. Think of being "bent ill" **(Bentyl)** you take this medicine from the IBS pain.

Hyoscyamine (Anaspaz)
High-uh-SIGH-uh-mean (AH-nuh-spaz)

The "an" prefix means against in medical terminology, so **Anaspaz** is against the IBS cramps and spasms.

CONSTIPATION – STOOL SOFTENER

Docusate Sodium (Colace)

DOCK-you-sate SEWED-e-um (CO-lace)

> **Docusate sodium** softens the stool. Patients use it with opioids like **morphine (Kadian)**. **Docusate** and "penetrate" rhyme, and **docusate sodium** works by helping water penetrate into the bowel. The brand **Colace** improves the <u>col</u>on's <u>pace</u>.

CONSTIPATION – OSMOTIC

Polyethylene Glycol (<u>PEG</u>) 3350 (MiraLax)
pa-Lee-ETH-ill-een GLY-call (MIR-uh-lacks)

> I remember **polyethylene glycol** because when my triplets were really young the triplets "**<u>poly</u>**" called "**<u>col</u>**" for me, "Daaaaaad! Can you wipe me?" **MiraLax** is the <u>Mira</u>cle <u>Lax</u>ative because it's a miracle how good you feel after taking it. By prescription, **Go-Lytely** is a 4-liter plastic bottle of **polyethylene glycol** used for colonoscopy examination preparation. There is nothing "lightly" about it.

CONSTIPATION – MISCELLANEOUS

Lubi<u>prost</u>one (Amitiza)
Lou-buh-PROS-tone (am-uh-TEE-zuh)

> I would also put **lubi<u>prost</u>one (Amitiza)** after **docusate sodium** and **polyethylene glycol** because it's a prescription item and would represent an escalation in the aggressiveness of treatment for constipation. While the "-prost-" stem indicates <u>prost</u>aglandin, it doesn't really help with immediate therapeutic recognition.

Antiemetic - Serotonin 5-HT₃ receptor antagonist

Ondan<u>setron</u> (Zofran, Zofran ODT)
on-DAN-se-tron (ZO-fran)

> The "setron" suffix will help you remember
> **ondansetron** is a serotonin 5-HT₃ receptor
> antagonist for preventing emesis. "O-D-T" stands
> for orally disintegrating tablet. It is a useful dosage
> form because it dissolves on the top of the tongue
> and requires no additional liquid. If you are good at
> word scrambles, **ondansetron** has every letter but
> the "i" in serotonin, a neurotransmitter, the majority
> of which is located in the GI tract.

Antiemetic - Phenothiazine

Prochlorperazine (Compazine)
pro-klor-PEAR-uh-zeen (KAM-puh-zeen)

> **Prochlorperazine (Compazine)** and **promethazine
> (Phenergan)** share the same first three letters, "p-r-
> o," and last five letters, "a-z-i-n-e." While this isn't a
> stem, both are phenothi<u>azine</u>s. By memorizing these
> two drugs in alphabetical order, you can use this
> similarity to recognize their comparable antiemetic
> function. Both happen to be available in suppository
> formulations as well

Promethazine (Phenergan)
pro-METH-uh-zeen (FEN-er-gan)

> **Promethazine** is an antihistamine sometimes used in
> liquid form with codeine. It also reduces nausea. In
> addition to oral, IM, and IV forms, **promethazine**

comes in a rectal suppository form if a patient can't take anything by the mouth (po).

III. GASTROINTESTINAL AUTOIMMUNE DISORDERS

Autoimmune diseases like Crohn's disease and ulcerative colitis (UC) occur when the body's immune system inappropriately attacks an area (or areas) of the body. Symptoms of UC include ulcerations and inflammation (-itis) in the colon. **Budesonide (Enterocort EC)** is a steroid that helps with inflammation. **Infliximab (Remicade)** blocks the tumor necrosis factor, alpha (TNF-alpha), to treat this disease.

ULCERATIVE COLITIS

Budesonide (Enterocort EC)
byou-DES-uh-nide (en-TER-uh-court)

> **Budesonide** has the son, s-o-n steroid infix, which isn't official but is useful. Your rear end is your bum which has the same first two letters b-u as budesonide, so you know where the medicine goes. Just like an enteral dosage form, the enter from **Enterocort EC**, means gastrointestinal tract and the cort, c-o-r-t means corticosteroid. So, in total a steroid for GI disorders.

Infliximab (Remicade)
in-FLIX-eh-mab (REM-eh-cade)

> **Infliximab** is a biologic agent, a genetically engineered protein. **Infliximab's** generic name should be broken up as inf + li +xi + mab. The "inf"

is a prefix that simply separates it from other similar drugs. The "li" stands for immunomodulator (the target). The "xi" stands for chimeric (the source, e.g., combining genetic material from a mouse, with genetic material from a human). The "x" might also refer to the Greek letter "chi," which looks like an x. The "mab" stands for monoclonal antibody. Conditions like ulcerative colitis can go into remission. **Remicade** is a "remission aide."

GASTROINTESTINAL DRUG QUIZ (LEVEL 1)

Classify these drugs by placing the corresponding drug class letter next to each medication. Try to underline the stems before you start and think about the brand name and function of each drug.

1. Calcium carbonate (Tums)
2. Nizatidine (Axid)
3. Docusate sodium (Colace)
4. Famotidine (Pepcid)
5. Esomeprazole (Nexium)
6. Loperamide (Imodium)
7. Magnesium hydroxide (Milk of Magnesia)
8. Infliximab (Remicade)
9. Omeprazole (Prilosec)
10. Ondansetron (Zofran)

Gastrointestinal drug classes:

A. Antacid
B. Anti-diarrheal
C. Anti-nausea
D. Constipation
E. H_2 blocker
F. Proton pump inhibitor
G. Ulcerative colitis

GASTROINTESTINAL DRUG QUIZ (LEVEL 2)

Classify these drugs by placing the corresponding drug class letter next to each medication. Try to underline the stems before you start and remember the brand name and function of each drug.

1. Bismuth Subsalicylate
2. Esomeprazole
3. Omeprazole
4. Polyethylene glycol
5. Promethazine
6. Calcium carbonate
7. Famotidine
8. Docusate sodium
9. Loperamide
10. Nizatidine

Gastrointestinal drug classes:

A. Antacid
B. Anti-diarrheal
C. Anti-nausea
D. Constipation
E. H$_2$ blocker
F. Proton pump inhibitor
G. Ulcerative colitis

PRACTICE EXAM PART 1
GASTROINTESTINAL

QUESTION G1. PEPTIC ULCER DISEASE CAUSES

A student asks how stomach ulcers come about. While there are many factors that can cause ulceration, one contributor to peptic ulcer disease might include:

a) Bicarbonate
b) Mucus
c) NSAIDs
d) Prostaglandins

Question G1. Peptic ulcer disease causes

A student asks how stomach ulcers come about. While there are many factors that can cause ulceration, one contributor to peptic ulcer disease might include:

a) Bicarbonate
b) Mucus
c) NSAIDs
d) Prostaglandins

Answer: C. **NSAIDs contribute to peptic ulcer disease** *as can Helicobacter pylori, an organism often found in ulcers.*

QUESTION G2. PEPTIC ULCER DISEASE DEFENSES

While the stomach is a hostile place for bacteria, there are protections built into the stomach to defend against peptic ulcer disease. A defender or protector against peptic ulcer disease might include:

a) Bicarbonate
b) *H. pylori*
c) NSAIDs
d) Pepsin

Question G2. Peptic ulcer disease defenses

While the stomach is a hostile place for bacteria, there are protections built into the stomach to defend against peptic ulcer disease. A defender or protector against peptic ulcer disease might include:

a) **Bicarbonate**
b) *H. pylori*
c) NSAIDs
d) Pepsin

Answer: A. Bicarbonate raises the pH protecting against ulceration. The pH scale is like a one-foot long ruler with 14 lines instead of 12. A "0" sits left for the most acidic compounds and a "14" sits right for the most basic or alkaline ones. 7, which is in the middle, is neutral. Stomach acid has a pH of 2; milk is 6; neutral is 7; and blood is 7.35. Why give dairy milk, which is slightly acidic, to calm an acidic stomach? Because 6 is more basic (alkaline) than 2. H. Pylori, a helicopter shaped organism, NSAIDs like ibuprofen and naproxen, and pepsin, a protein enzyme all can contribute to ulceration.

QUESTION G3: ANTACIDS

Sometimes, the easiest way to calm an upset stomach is to go to the over-the-counter pharmacy aisle. A patient complains of diarrhea and stomach indigestion; you suggest which antacid?

a) Esomeprazole
b) Famotidine
c) Calcium carbonate
d) Polyethylene glycol

Question G3: Antacids

Sometimes, the easiest way to calm an upset stomach is to go the over-the-counter pharmacy aisle. A patient complains of diarrhea and stomach indigestion; you suggest which antacid?

a) Esomeprazole
b) Famotidine
c) **Calcium carbonate**
d) Polyethylene glycol

Answer: C. Calcium carbonate (Tums) is the only antacid on the list and it's especially good for someone with diarrhea. Besides acting as an antacid, calcium carbonate can supplement calcium in a diet. Esomeprazole is a PPI, famotidine, an H-2 blocker, and polyethylene glycol, a laxative are all OTC, but none are antacids.

QUESTION G4. TIMING ACID REDUCERS

Taking a medicine at the right time can be critical to it working properly. When telling a patient when to take omeprazole, you say he or she should take it:

a) 1 to 3 hours after a meal
b) 1 to 3 hours before a meal
c) 30 minutes before a meal
d) With a meal

Question G4. Timing acid reducers

Taking a medicine at the right time can be critical to it working properly. When telling a patient when to take omeprazole, you say he or she should take it:

a) 1 to 3 hours after a meal
b) 1 to 3 hours before a meal
c) 30 minutes before a meal
d) With a meal

Answer: C. Omeprazole is best taken 30 minutes before a meal to prevent significant acid from forming in the first place. One might take an antacid 1 to 3 hours after a meal.

QUESTION G5. CHELATION INTERACTION

Drug interactions can be dangerous, but they can also completely inactivate the medicine. Chelation, or the binding of two medicines is one such reaction. A patient is on a fluoroquinolone antibiotic, you are concerned about chelation if you see this medicine in the chart:

a) Docusate sodium
b) Esomeprazole
c) Famotidine
d) Magnesium hydroxide

Question G5. Chelation interaction

Drug interactions can be dangerous, but they can also completely inactivate the medicine. Chelation, or the binding of two medicines is one such reaction. A patient is on a fluoroquinolone antibiotic, you are concerned about chelation if you see this medicine in the chart:

a) Docusate sodium
b) Esomeprazole
c) Famotidine
d) **Magnesium hydroxide**

Answer: D. Magnesium hydroxide (Milk of Magnesia) is an antacid and can bind or chelate with antibiotics like tetracyclines (Example: doxycycline, minocycline) or fluoroquinolones (Example: ciprofloxacin, levofloxacin). Milk of Magnesia looks like dairy milk, which can work similarly to an antacid in calming an acidic stomach. Put together the "milky texture" and the diarrhea of lactose intolerance to remember its laxative effect.

QUESTION G6. HISTAMINE-1 VS. HISTAMINE-2

We have different forms of histamine in our body, histamine-1 and histamine-2 for example. A histamine-2 receptor antagonist works well to treat:

a) Allergy symptoms
b) Constipation
c) Diarrhea
d) Nighttime GERD

Question G6. Histamine-1 vs. Histamine-2

We have different forms of histamine in our body, histamine-1 and histamine-2 for example. A histamine-2 receptor antagonist works well to treat:

a) Allergy symptoms
b) Constipation
c) Diarrhea
d) Nighttime GERD

Answer: D. Nighttime GERD would best respond to an H-2 blocker like famotidine (Pepcid). Pepcid contains "pep" from "peptic" and "pepsin" that relates to digestion, and "cid" from "acid." One student mentioned Pepsi, the soda, has a pH of 2.4, which is very acidic. She said it always gave her heartburn, so that's how she remembered Pepcid. Also, in soda pop, the "p-o-p" and Pepcid's "p-e-p" are very similar.

An H-1 blocker or antihistamine like loratadine would be appropriate for allergy symptoms.

QUESTION G7. DRUG STEMS

Often students who don't know there is an official list or accepted drug stems for non-proprietary medications (generics), make up stems using a few of the last letters in a drug name. But you know the proton pump inhibitor has the identifying stem:

a) -azole
b) -ole
c) -prazole
d) -zole

Question G7. Drug stems

Often students who don't know there is an official list or accepted drug stems for non-proprietary medications (generics), make up stems using a few of the last letters in a drug name. But you know the proton pump inhibitor has the identifying stem:

a) -azole
b) -ole
c) **-prazole**
d) -zole

Answer: C. -prazole is the official stem of a proton pump inhibitor (PPI); the other choices are incorrect endings you might find on electronic notecards. While esomeprazole (Nexium) and omeprazole (Prilosec) have the same ending "prazole," notice the only thing that separates omeprazole and esomeprazole is an "es." Many drugs have chemical structures that have mirror images called enantiomers. Instead of calling them right- and left-handed, we call them "R" and "S" from the Latin words rectus (right) and sinister (left). In this case, the "S" form is more active biologically. Putting an "s" in front of omeprazole would make "someprazole," which would be pronounced "some-prazole." Instead, the prefix "es" allows for a separation between the "S" sound and the compound name, as a chemist would pronounce it.

QUESTION G8. EFFECTS ON pH

Some medications raise pH and others lower pH to affect their response. A proton pump inhibitor has this effect on pH:

a) Lowers
b) Moving ph closer to 1
c) Moving ph closer to 2
d) Raises

Question G8. Effects on pH

Some medications raise pH and others lower pH to affect their response. A proton pump inhibitor has this effect on pH:

a) Lowers
b) Moving ph closer to 1
c) Moving ph closer to 2
d) Raises

Answer: D. Raises. The pH goes up as there is less acid and makes the stomach more alkaline.

QUESTION G9. NSAID INDUCED ULCER

The cause of peptic ulcer disease is important in knowing which medication to give. With NSAID-induced ulcer treatment, we expect to see:

a) Acid reducers alone
b) One antibiotic and one acid reducer
c) One antibiotic and two acid reducers
d) Two antibiotics and one acid reducer

Question G9. NSAID induced ulcer

The cause of peptic ulcer disease is important in knowing which medication to give. With NSAID-induced ulcer treatment, we expect to see:

a) **Acid reducers alone**
b) One antibiotic and one acid reducer
c) One antibiotic and two acid reducers
d) Two antibiotics and one acid reducer

Answer: A. Acid reducers alone would be appropriate therapy with NSAIDS. If H. Pylori was the culprit, we would expect to see two antibiotics or more and one acid reducer.

QUESTION G10. *H. PYLORI* INDUCED ULCER

The cause of peptic ulcer disease is important in knowing which medication to give. With *Helicobacter pylori*-induced ulcer treatment, we expect to see:

a) Acid reducers alone
b) One antibiotic and one acid reducer
c) One antibiotic and two acid reducers
d) Two antibiotics and one acid reducer

Question G10. *H. pylori* induced ulcer

The cause of peptic ulcer disease is important in knowing which medication to give. With *Helicobacter pylori*-induced ulcer treatment, we expect to see:

a) Acid reducers alone
b) One antibiotic and one acid reducer
c) One antibiotic and two acid reducers
d) **Two antibiotics and one acid reducer**

Answer: D. If H. Pylori was the culprit, we would expect to see two antibiotics or more and one acid reducer.

QUESTION G11. NON-DRUG PUD TREATMENT

While medications are the mainstay of treatment for peptic ulcer disease, there are non-drug options for treatment. All of the following are non-drug treatments for peptic ulcer disase except:

a) Eat 5-6 small meals daily
b) Avoid smoking
c) Continue NSAIDs for pain
d) Avoid alcohol and caffeine

Question G11. Non-drug PUD treatment

While medications are the mainstay of treatment for peptic ulcer disease, there are non-drug options for treatment. All of the following are non-drug treatments for peptic ulcer disase except:

a) Eat 5-6 small meals daily
b) Avoid smoking
c) **Continue NSAIDs for pain**
d) Avoid alcohol and caffeine

Answer: C. One would stop NSAIDs to try to reduce the chance of an ulcer. Eating 5-6 small meals a day, avoiding smoking, alcohol and caffeine may help as well.

QUESTION G12. LAXATIVE EFFECTS

Patients might come to you asking for constipation relief with the "strongest thing you got." However, there are different classes of laxatives for different effects. A stimulant constipation treatment would include:

a) Docusate sodium
b) Polyethylene glycol
c) Psyllium
d) Senna

Question G12. Laxative effects

Patients might come to you asking for constipation relief with the "strongest thing you got." However, there are different classes of laxatives for different effects. A stimulant constipation treatment would include:

a) Docusate sodium
b) Polyethylene glycol
c) Psyllium
d) Senna

Answer: D. Senna is a stimulant laxative. Docusate is a stool softener, polyethylene glycol is an osmotic, and psyllium is fiber or bulk forming.

QUESTION G13. LAXATIVE CLASSES

A laxative class similar to dietary fiber that can take up to three days to produce a bowel movement is:

a) Docusate sodium
b) Polyethylene glycol
c) Psyllium
d) Senna

Question G13. Laxative classes

A laxative class similar to dietary fiber that can take up to three days to produce a bowel movement is:

a) Docusate sodium
b) Polyethylene glycol
c) Psyllium
d) Senna

Answer: C. Psyllium is similar to dietary fiber. Docusate sodium softens the stool. Patients use it with opioids like morphine (Kadian). Docusate and "penetrate" rhyme, and docusate sodium works by helping water penetrate into the bowel. The brand Colace improves the colon's pace. Polyethylene glycol is an osmotic and senna is a stimulant laxative

QUESTION G14. PEDIATRICS AND CONSTIPATION

A patient says his prescriber gave him a recommendation for the laxative that's generally gentle and safe for children and that's in a container with a purple cap. Which medicine is he talking about?

a) Bismuth subsalicylate
b) Magnesium hydroxide
c) Polyethylene glycol (GoLytely)
d) Polyethylene glycol (MiraLAX)

Question G14. Pediatrics and constipation

A patient says his prescriber gave him a recommendation for the laxative that's generally gentle and safe for children and that's in a container with a purple cap. Which medicine is he talking about?

a) Bismuth subsalicylate
b) Magnesium hydroxide
c) Polyethylene glycol (GoLytely)
d) Polyethylene glycol (MiraLAX)

Answer: D. Polyethylene glycol (MiraLAX) is the Miracle Laxative because how good you feel after taking it is a miracle. It's not uncommon for a patient to ask for a medicine by describing what the medicine looks like when the name is complicated. Bismuth subsalicylate or Pepto-bismol is usually in a pink bottle, magnesium hydroxide (Milk of Magnesia) is in a blue bottle, and polyethylene glycol (GoLytely) is a gallon jug for bowel prep.

QUESTION G15. OTC VS. PRESCRIPTION

Sometimes patients from other countries struggle to find medicines because in their country the pharmacist could give them certain medicines without a prescription. A patient tells you his diarrhea is so bad that he needs a prescription medicine. Which medicine was he likely taking?

a) Bismuth subsalicylate
b) Diphenoxylate / atropine
c) Famotidine
d) Loperamide

Question G15. OTC vs. prescription

Sometimes patients from other countries struggle to find medicines because in their country the pharmacist could give them certain medicines without a prescription. A patient tells you his diarrhea is so bad, he needs a prescription medicine. Which medicine was he likely taking?

a) Bismuth subsalicylate
b) Diphenoxylate / atropine
c) Famotidine
d) Loperamide

Answer: B. Diphenoxylate / atropine (Lomotil) is a prescription antidiarrheal with a DEA schedule V rating. Diphenoxylate with atropine represents an increase in the aggressiveness of treatment from OTC to prescription. The brand name Lomotil spells out "low motility" for slowing down diarrhea. The atropine is there to prevent someone from crushing the diphenoxylate and injecting it illicitly. Bismuth subsalicylate is for indigestion and diarrhea, famotidine is an H-2 blocker for acid, and loperamide is an antidiarrheal. (GoLytely) is a gallon jug for bowel prep.

QUESTION G16. CHILDREN'S SAFETY

When talking to a parent about a pediatric patient and Pepto Children's, which of the following would be a true statement?

a) Bismuth subsalicylate is the active ingredient for children
b) Calcium carbonate is the active ingredient for children
c) It can cause Reye's syndrome
d) It has a laxative effect

Question G16. Children's safety

When talking to a parent about a pediatric patient and Pepto Children's, which of the following would be a true statement?

a) Bismuth subsalicylate is the active ingredient for children
b) Calcium carbonate is the active ingredient for children
c) It can cause Reye's syndrome
d) It has a laxative effect

Answer: B. Calcium carbonate is the active ingredient in Pepto Children's while bismuth subsalicylate is the active ingredient in Pepto-bismol. The salicylate component can cause Reye's syndrome in children and bismuth is an antidiarrheal rather than a laxative. The "b" in bismuth subsalicylate reminds students of the black tongue and black stool that some patients experience as side effects. (Note: This discoloration is harmless.) Pepto looks like peptic, which has to do with digestion.

QUESTION G17. INFECTIOUS DIARRHEA

A patient knows he will be going into an area with poor water quality and that he might have to take a prescription medicine on his travels. Which medication would best treat infectious diarrhea?

a) Bismuth subsalicylate
b) Ciprofloxacin
c) Diphenoxylate / atropine
d) Loperamide

Question G17. Infectious diarrhea

A patient knows he will be going into an area with poor water quality and that he might have to take a prescription medicine on his travels. Which medication would best treat infectious diarrhea?

 a) Bismuth subsalicylate
 b) Ciprofloxacin
 c) Diphenoxylate / atropine
 d) Loperamide

Answer: B. Ciprofloxacin is an antibiotic one might use for infectious diarrhea. The quinolone stem is "-oxacin," but fluoroquinolones have the "-fl-" infix also. One student remembered quinolones are for UTIs because Dr. Quinn, Medicine Woman, is female. Women get proportionally more UTIs than men do. By cutting the "–floxacin" stem from the generic name ciprofloxacin, the manufacturer made the brand name, Cipro. While bismuth subsalicylate, diphenoxylate / atropine, and loperamide are all antidiarrheals, none would eliminate a bacterial infection.

QUESTION G18. TYPES OF EMESES

When treating nausea and vomiting we have to be cognizant of three types of emeses. Which of the following is not a type of emesis that a patient might have?

a) Anterograde
b) Anticipatory
c) Acute
d) Delayed

Question G18. Types of emeses

When treating nausea and vomiting we have to be cognizant of three types of emeses. Which of the following is not a type of emesis that a patient might have?

a) **Anterograde**
b) Anticipatory
c) Acute
d) Delayed

Answer: A. Anterograde refers to a type of amnesia where a patient might have trouble forming memories. Anticipatory nausea is triggered by a memory of severe nausea from a previous dose. Acute happens a few minutes after giving a medication. Delayed emesis would happen over a day later. It appears 48 to 72 hours after chemotherapy.

QUESTION G19. SEROTONIN ACRONYMS

While students can often remember that 5-HT is a way of representing serotonin, often the numbers and mechanism of action can get mixed up. We believe ondansetron's mechanism of action is as a:

a) 5-HT1 agonist
b) 5-HT1 antagonist
c) 5-HT3 agonist
d) 5-HT3 antagonist

Question G19. Serotonin acronyms

While students can often remember that 5-HT is a way of representing serotonin, often the numbers and mechanism of action can get mixed up. We believe ondansetron's mechanism of action is as a:

a) 5-HT1 agonist
b) 5-HT1 antagonist
c) 5-HT3 agonist
d) 5-HT3 antagonist

Answer: D. 5HT-3 antagonist represents ondansetron's mechanism of action. The "setron" suffix will help you remember ondansetron is a serotonin 5-HT3 receptor antagonist for preventing emesis. "O-D-T" stands for orally disintegrating tablet. It is a useful dosage form because it dissolves on the top of the tongue and requires no additional liquid. If you are good at word scrambles, ondansetron has every letter but the "i" in serotonin, a neurotransmitter, the majority of which is located in the GI tract. Sumatriptan, a migraine medicine works as a 5-HT1 agonist.

QUESTION G20. INFLAMMATORY BOWEL DISEASE

There are many treatments, none of which are curative for inflammatory bowel disease. Which of the following medication classes best demonstrates in which class infliximab would belong?

a) 5-aminosalicylates
b) Glucocorticoids
c) Immunomodulators
d) Immunosuppressants

Question G20. Inflammatory bowel disease

There are many treatments, none of which are curative for inflammatory bowel disease. Which of the following medication classes best demonstrates in which class infliximab would belong?

a) 5-aminosalicylates
b) Glucocorticoids
c) **Immunomodulators**
d) Immunosuppressants

Answer: C. Immunomodulators include infliximab. Infliximab is a biologic agent, a genetically engineered protein. Infliximab's generic name should be broken up as inf + li +xi + mab. The "inf" is a prefix that separates it from similar drugs. The "li" stands for immunomodulator (the target). The "xi" stands for chimeric (the source, e.g., combining genetic material from a mouse, with a human's). The "x" might also refer to the Greek letter "chi," which looks like an x. The "mab" stands for monoclonal antibody. Conditions like ulcerative colitis can go into remission. Remicade is a "remission aide." Examples of 5-aminosalicylates are sulfasalazine and mesalamine. Glucocorticoids can include hydrocortisone and dexamethasone. Immunosuppressants are azathioprine, cyclosporine, and methotrexate.

CHAPTER 2
MUSCULOSKELETAL

I. NSAIDs AND PAIN

Non-steroidal anti-inflammatory drugs (NSAIDs) (pronounced *EN-SAIDs*) contrast with the steroidal medications used to treat inflammation. The NSAIDs **aspirin (Ecotrin)** and **ibuprofen (Advil, Motrin)** [taken up to four times daily] and **naproxen (Aleve)** [taken twice daily] are available over-the-counter and are for sporadic or mild pain. **Meloxicam (Mobic)** [once daily] isn't OTC and has the longest half-life. *Analgesics* relieve pain. *Antipyretics* reduce fever. NSAIDs are both.

NSAIDs like **ibuprofen** can close an arterial shunt (*patent ductus arteriosus*) in a preemie. Our newborn daughter had this condition. I watched a YouTube video on the surgery to close the shunt and it took only five minutes, but surgery on any NICU neonate runs a great risk. We were thankful a simple NSAID closed the shunt.

A regular pharmacy question is when to use **acetaminophen (Tylenol)** and when to use an **NSAID**. If the patient has inflammation, prescribers prefer NSAIDs, as analgesics like **acetaminophen** will not help. However, if the patient has pain or fever, then either is appropriate. Generally, NSAIDs are not used for pregnant patients, but **acetaminophen (Tylenol)** can be.

Excedrin Migraine contains three drugs: **aspirin** for pain and inflammation, **acetaminophen** for pain, and **caffeine** as a potent vasoconstrictor. It narrows swollen brain vessels.

Common NSAIDs block both cyclooxygenase (COX) -1 and -2 to minimize inflammatory processes. COX-1 blockade reduces inflammation in the body and, unfortunately, the body's natural protection of the stomach lining. Note that a selective COX-2 inhibitor, like **celecoxib (Celebrex)** does not block the protective effect of COX-1 against stomach ulcers and this is why it's supposed to be a better choice.

OTC ANALGESICS – NSAIDS

Aspirin [ASA] (Ecotrin)
AS-per-in (ECK-oh-trin)

> The acronym for aspirin, "ASA," comes from the chemical name: AcetylSalicylicAcid. **Ecotrin** is enteric-coated aspirin.

Ibuprofen (Advil, Motrin)
eye-byou-PRO-fin (ADD-vil, MO-trin)

> Many students try to say that **ibuprofen** and **naproxen** both end with "en." However, many drugs end with "e-n," so that won't help in a large multiple-choice exam. A better mnemonic is to notice that "-profen" from **ibuprofen** is a recognized stem and differs from "proxen" in **naproxen** by only one letter.

Naproxen (Aleve)
nap-ROCKS-in (uh-LEAVE)

> While **naproxen** has no formal stem, a student came up with a mnemonic for the brand name: **Aleve will** alleviate pain from strains and sprains.

OTC Analgesic – Non-narcotic

Acetaminophen [APAP] (Tylenol)
uh-seat-uh-MIN-no-fin (TIE-len-all)

> The brand **Tylenol**, generic **acetaminophen**, and acronym **APAP** all come from the chemical name:
>
> N-ace<u>t</u>yl-para-amino-ph<u>en</u>ol (**Tylenol**)
> N-<u>ace</u>tyl-para-<u>amino</u>-ph<u>en</u>ol (**Acetaminophen**)
> N-<u>A</u>cetyl-<u>P</u>ara-<u>A</u>mino-<u>P</u>henol (**APAP**)

OTC Migraine – NSAID / Non-narcotic analgesic

Aspirin / Acetaminophen / Caffeine (Excedrin Migraine)
AS-per-in / uh-seat-uh-MIN-oh-fin / KAF-feen (ecks-SAID-rin)

> Most students remember **Excedrin Migraine** by the rationale for the combination of **ASA / APAP / caffeine**: inflammation / analgesia / vasoconstriction.

Rx Migraine – Narcotic and Non-narcotic analgesic

Butalbital / Acetaminophen / Caffeine (Fioricet)
BYOU-tall-bih-tall / uh-seat-uh-MIN-oh-fin / KAF-feen (FEE-or-ih-set)

> Adding **butalbital**, a barbiturate, to **acetaminophen** and **caffeine** in **Fioricet** provides an escalation from the OTC **aspirin / acetaminophen / caffeine** combination in **Excedrin Migraine**. I pair those two drugs in my mind to help remember their therapeutic function.

71

RX ANALGESICS – NSAIDS

Diclofenac sodium extended release (Voltaren XR)
die-KLO-fuh-nak SEW-dee-um (VOL-tuh-ruhn)

> **Diclofenac** is a generic name derived from its chemical structure 2-(2,6-dichloranilino) phenylacetic acid with a change from "p-h" to "f" in the middle. There is a Voltaren Topical Gel that provides arthritis pain relief that contains diclofenac as the active ingredient.

Etodolac (Lodine)
eh-TOE-duh-lack (LOW-dean)

> **Etodolac** (**Lodine**) shares the same generic stem, "ac" tying it to diclofenac.

Indomethacin (Indocin)
in-doe-MEH-thuh-sin (IN-doe-sin)

> The manufacturers of **indomethacin** simply removed the middle "metha" to get the brand name **Indocin**.

Meloxicam (Mobic)
mel-OX-eh-kam (MO-bik)

> The "-icam" suffix in the generic name **meloxicam** lets you know it's an NSAID. A student used the "bic" in **Mobic** to remember it treats "big" swelling.

Nabumetone (Relafen)
nah-BYOU-mih-tone (REL-uh-fin)

Nabumetone's brand name **Relafen** sounds a little like getting pain <u>rel</u>ief with an "<u>en</u>-said."

RX ANALGESICS – NSAIDs – COX-2 INHIBITOR

Cele<u>coxib</u> (Celebrex)
sell-eh-COCKS-ib (SELL-eh-breks)

The "–coxib" suffix lets you know celecoxib is a selective COX-2 inhibitor. The commercials for **Celebrex** talk about <u>celebra</u>ting relief from inflammatory conditions. Regular NSAIDs like **ibuprofen** and **naproxen** inhibit both COX-1 and COX-2, causing the stomach distress so commonly caused by drugs in the NSAID class. **Celebrex** causes less GI irritation due to its lack of COX-1 inhibition.

II. OPIOIDS AND NARCOTICS

Opioids relieve pain, but have addiction potential. The DEA (Drug Enforcement Agency) categorizes the addictive potential of medications using a drug scheduling system.

Schedule I drugs are illegal substances and have no medical value, such as **heroin.**

Schedule II drugs are potentially addicting, such as the individual drugs **fentanyl (Duragesic, Sublimaze) and morphine (Kadian),** and the combination products **hydrocodone / APAP (Vicodin)** and **oxycodone / APAP (Percocet).**

Schedule III drugs are less addicting and include **acetaminophen / codeine (Tylenol with codeine).**

Schedule IV drugs include some sedative-hypnotics (sleeping pills) such as **zolpidem** (**Ambien)** and mixed opioid analgesics like **tramadol (Ultram)**.

Schedule V drugs are often cough medicines like **guaifenesin / codeine (Cheratussin AC)** that include codeine, but not **codeine** as a drug alone.

An opioid side effect is pinpoint pupils called miosis. A student remembered this by noticing that the words "opioid" and "miosis" both have two little dots over the two i's that look like pinpoint pupils.

OPIOID ANALGESICS – SCHEDULE II

Morphine (Kadian, MS Contin)
MORE-feen (KAY-dee-en, EM-ES KON-tin)

> The generic name **morphine** comes from the ancient Greek god of dreams, Morpheus. **Kadian** might come from cir**cadian** (the twenty-four-hour cycle) because **Kadian** is an extended-release morphine formulation. **MS Contin** stands for **m**orphine **s**ulfate **contin**uous release.

Fentanyl (Duragesic, Sublimaze)
FEN-ta-nil (dur-uh-GEE-zic, SUB-leh-maze)

> **Fentanyl** is troubling because it's dosed in micrograms, not milligrams. When it was time to give our three-month-old preemie **fentanyl** after her pyloric valve stenosis surgery in the Neonatal Intensive Care Unit (NICU), I made sure to check the calculated dose. **Duragesic** is a long **dura**tion anal**gesic** and comes in a patch that provides relief for 72 hours. **Sublimaze** is an injectable form of **fentanyl**.

Hydrocodone / Acetaminophen (Vicodin)
high-droe-CO-done / uh-seat-uh-MIN-no-fin (VIE-co-din)

> **Hydrocodone** and **oxycodone** differ slightly in chemical structure. **Oxycodone** has one more oxygen than **hydrocodone**. **Oxycodone/APAP** gets its name from the first three letters of *oxy*gen. **Hydrocodone/APAP** has only one hydrogen and gets its name from the first five letters of *hydro*gen. The "c-o-d-i-n" in **Vicodin** looks like **codeine,** just drop two e's from codeine, so you can remember they are related.

Hydrocodone / Chlorpheniramine (Tussionex)
high-droe-CO-done / klor-feh-NEER-uh-meen (TUSS-ee-uh-necks)

> **Tussionex** is a pineapple-flavored liquid anti<u>tuss</u>ive, hence the brand name. Chlorpheniramine is a drying first-generation antihistamine for those post-nasal drip coughs.

Hydrocodone / Ibuprofen (Vicoprofen)
high-droe-CO-done / eye-byou-PRO-fin (VIE-co-PRO-fin)

> **Vicoprofen** is like <u>**Vicodin**</u>, but with **ibuprofen** instead of **acetaminophen**. Therefore, the manufacturer replaced the "i-b-u" from **ibuprofen** with "V-i-c-o" of **Vicodin**.

Methadone (Dolophine)
MEH-thuh-done (DOW-luh-feen)

> A **methadone** clinic is one that tries to get patients off of opioids. The brand name **Dolophine** combines "dolo" from dolor in Spanish meaning pain and

"phine" from morphine to help you remember the connection to pain or morphine addiction.

Oxycodone (OxyIR, Oxycontin)
ak-see-CO-done-CO-done (AK-see EYE-are, AK-see-KAN-tin)

> **Oxycodone** by itself comes in an immediate release form, **OxyIR**, and an extended-release form, **OxyContin**. The "c-o-n-t-i-n" means <u>contin</u>uous release. Many people mispronounce this as oxy-cotton, using a word they are familiar with.

Oxycodone/Acetaminophen (Percocet)
ox-e-CO-done / uh-seat-uh-MIN-no-fin (PER-coe-set)

> The "cet" in **Percocet** comes from a<u>cet</u>aminophen. Some students use that "codone" and "codeine" look a little alike to remember the similarity, but this is not a true stem and **Percocet** does not contain codeine. Drug companies add **acetaminophen** as a mild analgesic.

Opioid analgesics – Schedule III

Acetaminophen/Codeine (Tylenol/Codeine, Tylenol #3)
uh-seat-uh-MIN-no-fin with CO-dean
(TIE-len-all with CO-dean, TIE-len-all NUM-ber three)

> I am not sure why, but when you say the generic name of **Vicodin**, you say "**hydrocodone with acetaminophen**," but when you talk about **codeine**, the order is reversed. It's phrased as "**acetaminophen with codeine**" (Tylenol w/codeine). Students seem to remember both because of the reverse / opposite order. The "#3" in

Tylenol #3 refers to the amount of codeine in combination. For example:

Tylenol #2 15 mg codeine / 300 mg acetaminophen
Tylenol #3 30 mg codeine / 300 mg acetaminophen
Tylenol #4 60 mg codeine / 300 mg acetaminophen

MIXED-OPIOID RECEPTOR ANALGESIC – SCHEDULE IV

Tramadol (Ultram)
TRA-muh-doll (ULL-tram)

> **Tramadol** only weakly affects opioid receptors. For this reason, the DEA did not classify **tramadol** as a controlled substance until 2014. The "–adol" stem indicates that it's a mixed opioid analgesic. Many students have thought of "tram wreck" and "train wreck" as a way to remember that **Ultram** is used for pain.

Tramadol / Acetaminophen (Ultracet)
TRA-muh-doll / uh-seat-uh-MIN-no-fin (ULL-truh-set)

> **Tramadol** with **acetaminophen (Ultracet)** follows **tramadol** by itself. The manufacturer took the brand name **Ultram** (for **tramadol** alone), dropped the "m" and added "acet" from **acetaminophen**.

OPIOID ANTAGONIST

Naloxone (Narcan)
nah-LOX-own (NAR-can)

> **Naloxone** is an opioid receptor antagonist used in opioid overdose situations. Often it's in the L-E-A-N

acronym of emergency medicines **lidocaine,
epinephrine, atropine**, and **naloxone**. The "nal-"
stem in **naloxone** indicates it's an opioid receptor
antagonist, but the brand name **Narcan** also hints at
a narcotic antagonist.

Buprenorphine / Naloxone (Suboxone) [CIII]
Byou-prih-NOR-feen (sub-AWK-sewn)

> Patients use **buprenorphine / naloxone (Suboxone)**
> like **methadone** to help detox from opiate addiction.
> The **naloxone** is there to keep patients from
> crushing the drug and injecting it.

III. HEADACHES AND MIGRAINES

Common OTC drugs for headache and migraine include
the NSAIDs like **aspirin (Ecotrin), ibuprofen (Advil,
Motrin), naproxen (Aleve)**, and the combination **ASA /
APAP / Caffeine (Excedrin Migraine)** reviewed earlier.

Sometimes severe migraines require drugs in the 5-HT_1
receptor agonist class, such as **eletriptan (Relpax)** and
sumatriptan (Imitrex) that work by activating receptors
that reduce the swelling associated with migraines. We call
them **triptans** because those two syllables are easier to say
than "5-hydroxytryptamine receptor agonists" is.

It's important to contrast the terms **agonist** and **antagonist**
as opposites. An agonist is a drug that activates a receptor
while an antagonist blocks the receptor. There is no reason
to *produce* migraines, but a 5-HT_1 receptor *antagonist* would
likely cause a headache, whereas the corresponding agonist
alleviates headaches. One student thought of agonists as
when she first stepped on an elliptical exercise machine and
it awakened the screen. She thought of antagonist as her

own excuses why she could not work out. Another metaphor you will often see is that of dating. There are some funny videos on YouTube about agonism versus antagonism. The agonist is usually someone who wants to get a date and the antagonist tries to block the suitor.

5-HT$_1$ RECEPTOR AGONIST

Eletriptan (Relpax)
el-eh-TRIP-tan (rel-PAKS)

> Remember **eletriptan** from its suffix "–triptan" so you can recognize the many other medications in the triptan class. The brand name **Relpax** combines "pax," the Latin word for "peace" and "Rel," for "relief." I often confused whether this was an agonist or antagonist, but use the "agony" of a migraine to remember triptans as agonists.

Sumatriptan (Imitrex)
Sue-ma-TRIP-tan (IM-eh-treks)

> Remember **sumatriptan** from its suffix "–triptan." Students say it "trips up" a headache. Also, the "i-m" in the brand name **Imitrex** reminds you there is an intramuscular (IM) form for patients who have such a severe migraine that they can't take anything by mouth.

IV. DMARDs AND RHEUMATOID ARTHRITIS

DMARD stands for **D**isease-**M**odifying **A**nti-**R**heumatic **D**rug, which means it works against *rheumatoid arthritis*, an autoimmune disorder. These drugs reduce the progression of the disease as opposed to the treatment of *osteoarthritis*, a condition in which the body has worn down and the joints are inflamed.

Both conditions respond to NSAID anti-inflammatories such as **ibuprofen (Advil, Motrin)** or **aspirin (Ecotrin)**. Additionally, glucocorticoids, such as **prednisone (Deltasone),** can further help reduce inflammation in the joints.

Prescribers use special immune-suppressing drugs called DMARDs like **methotrexate (Rheumatrex), abatacept (Orencia)** and **etanercept (Enbrel)** for rheumatoid arthritis.

DMARDs

Methotrexate (Rheumatrex)
meth-oh-TREKS-ate (ROOM-uh-treks)

> One student came up with "Meth o T-Rex ate the rheumatic inflammate." The "rheuma" in the brand name **Rheumatrex** reminds you it relieves rheumatoid arthritis.

Abatacept (Orencia)
uh-BAT-uh-sep" (or-EN-see-uh)

> **Abatacept** and **etanercept** have complex stems. The "-ta-" infix in **abatacept** means it's going after T-cell receptors and the suffix "–cept" means that it's a re**cept**or molecule, either native or modified.

Etanercept (Enbrel)
eh-ta-NER-sept (EN-brell)

> Learn **etanercept** and **abatacept** from the suffix "–cept" with the added sub-stem "-tacept" or "-nercept" respectively. The "-ner-" infix in **etanercept**

point out that it goes after tumor <u>necr</u>osis factor receptors.

V. Osteoporosis

Don't confuse *osteoarthritis*, a joint disease, with *osteoporosis*, a thinning in bone tissue density. Drugs for osteoarthritis include the NSAIDs. Drugs for osteoporosis build bone back up. Humans' bones grow slowly. Therefore, drugs like **alendronate (Fosamax)** can be given weekly, and **ibandronate (Boniva)** can be given monthly. A special precaution for patients using **alendronate** is to not lie down for 30 minutes after taking the medication; for **ibandronate**, it's 60 minutes.

Bisphosphonates

Alen<u>dronate</u> (Fosamax)
uh-LEN-dro-nate (FA-seh-max)

> Memorize **alendronate** as a calcium metabolism regulator from its "-dronate" stem. Students like to remember that "drone" rhymes with bone. Many students have said that the brand name **Fosamax** looks like "fossil."

Iban<u>dronate</u> (Boniva)
eh-BAND-row-nate" (bo-KNEE-vuh)

> Again, the "–dronate" suffix should be your key to the drug class, but having the first three letters of bone in the brand name **Boniva** helps. The generic **ibandronate** contains all the letters in **Boniva** except the "v."

Rise<u>dronate</u> (Actonel)

rih-SED-druh-nate (AK-tuh-nell)

> **Risedronate (Actonel)** is simply another
> bisphosphonate that you can recognize from the "-
> dronate" stem. Actonel is "<u>act</u>ing on <u>bone</u>."

VI. SELECTIVE ESTROGEN RECEPTOR MODULATOR (SERM)

Raloxifene (Evista)
ruh-LAWK-suh-feen (ee-VIS-tuh)

> We classify the <u>s</u>elective <u>e</u>strogen <u>r</u>eceptor
> <u>m</u>odulator (SERM) **raloxifene (Evista)** as an
> antiestrogen by its "–ifene" stem.

VII. MUSCLE RELAXANTS

The DEA doesn't schedule **cyclobenzaprine (Flexeril)**, but
does schedule **diazepam (Valium)** as C-IV. Both drugs
provide muscle relaxation and relief from muscle spasms.

Baclofen (Lioresal)
BAK-low-fen (Lee-OR-ih-sal)

> **Baclofen** has the word "back" in it, a place where
> many find a pulled muscle. And **Lioresal** always
> made me think "lie or sit down" when you have
> muscle pain. It's also for multiple sclerosis (MS).

Carisoprodol (Soma)
kuh-rih-suh-PRO-doll (SEW-muh)

Soma sounds like <u>som</u>nolence (sleepiness), and if you are a literature nerd like me, this drug was a hallucinogen in Aldous Huxley's 1932 book, *Brave New World*.

Metaxalone (Skelaxin)
meh-TAK-suh-lone (SKUH-lack-sin)

Skelaxin alludes to "<u>skel</u>etal rel<u>axin</u>'."

Methocarbamol (Robaxin)
meth-uh-KAR-buh-mol (row-BACKS-in)

Robaxin and rel<u>axin</u>' go together.

Tizanidine (Zanaflex)
tie-ZAN-ih-dean (ZAN-uh-flecks)

Zanaflex ends with "flex" for increased <u>flex</u>ibility.

Cyclobenzaprine (Flexeril)
sigh-clo-BENDS-uh-preen (FLEX-er-ill)

Cyclobenzaprine helps you get bending again. **Flexeril** improves flexibility.

Di<u>aze</u>pam (Valium)
dye-AY-zeh-pam" (VAL-e-um)

Diazepam and benzo**diazep**ine, diazepam's drug class, have similar letters. **Val**erian root is an herbal remedy for anxiety; some think of **Valium** as relaxing both anxiety and muscles in the same way.

VIII. Gout

Gout is an acute inflammatory arthritis we treat acutely (right away) with an NSAID like **ibuprofen** (**Advil**, **Motrin**) We can treat also treat gout prophylactically by reducing uric acid, a major component in the crystals that cause the gouty pain. Drugs that alter uric acid levels include **allopurinol (Zyloprim)** and **febuxostat (Uloric)**.

Colchicine (Colcrys)
KOWL-chu-seen (COAL-Chris)

> **Colchicine (Colcrys)** relieves an acute gouty attack, so I put that before the uric acid reducers that treat chronic increased uric acid. The "crys" in **Colcrys** sounds like the painful gouty <u>crys</u>tals that often form in the big toe. Google "gouty crystal" images and you'll see that they look like needles.

Uric acid reducers

Allopurinol (Zyloprim)
a-loe-PURE-in-all (ZY-low-prim)

> Within **allopurinol**, you can see "uri," which corresponds to the uric acid the medication reduces. You can also remember this is an anti-arthritic by thinking of the joints as becoming "all-pure-and-all."

Febu<u>x</u>ostat (Uloric)
fe-BUCKS-oh-stat (YOU-lore-ick)

> The "-xostat" stem in **febuxostat** indicates a <u>x</u>anthine <u>o</u>xidase inhibitor that prevents uric acid from forming. The "x" and "o" in the generic name

match xanthine oxidase. The brand name **Uloric** looks like "U" "lower" "uric acid."

Probenecid (Benemid)
PRO-ben-uh-sid (BEN-uh-mid)

You can see the end of uric acid in **probenecid** to help you remember its use. **Benemid**, probenecid, and benefit share the ben, b-e-n to connect those as benefitting gout patients.

MUSCULOSKELETAL DRUG QUIZ (LEVEL 1)

Classify these drugs by placing the corresponding drug class letter next to each medication. Try to underline the stems before you start and think about the brand name and function of each drug.

1. Acetaminophen (Tylenol)
2. Alendronate (Fosamax)
3. ASA/APAP/Caffeine (Excedrin)
4. Febuxostat (Uloric)
5. Etanercept (Enbrel)
6. Fentanyl (Duragesic)
7. Hydrocodone / APAP (Vicodin)
8. Ibuprofen (Advil, Motrin)
9. Celecoxib (Celebrex)
10. Sumatriptan (Imitrex)

Musculoskeletal Drug Classes:

A. 5-HT$_1$ receptor agonist
B. Anti-gout
C. Bisphosphonate
D. DMARD
E. Non-narcotic analgesic – single
F. Non-narcotic analgesic combo - headache
G. NSAID not COX-2 selective
H. NSAID COX-2 selective
I. Opioid analgesic

MUSCULOSKELETAL DRUG QUIZ (LEVEL 2)

Classify these drugs by placing the corresponding drug class letter next to each medication. Try to underline the stems before you start and remember the brand name and function of each drug.

1. Methotrexate
2. Morphine
3. Abatacept
4. Naproxen
5. Febuxostat
6. Ibandronate
7. Allopurinol
8. Aspirin
9. Alendronate
10. APAP/Codeine

Musculoskeletal Drug Classes:

A. 5-HT$_1$ receptor agonist
B. Anti-gout
C. Bisphosphonate
D. DMARD
E. Non-narcotic analgesic - single
F. Non-narcotic analgesic combo - headache
G. NSAID not COX-2 selective
H. NSAID COX-2 selective
I. Opioid analgesic

PRACTICE EXAM PART 2
MUSCULOSKELETAL

QUESTION M1. CYCLOOXYGENASE (COX-1, COX-2)

Cyclooxygenase, an enzyme important in prostaglandin formation, abbreviated COX, has a form that we colloquially refer to as either good COX or bad COX. Which cyclooxygenase is the "bad COX"?

a) COX-1
b) COX-2
c) COX-3
d) COX-4

Question M1. Cyclooxygenase (Cox-1, Cox-2)

Cyclooxygenase, an enzyme important in prostaglandin formation, abbreviated COX, has a form that we colloquially refer to as good COX and bad COX. Which cyclooxygenase is the "bad COX?"

a) COX-1
b) COX-2
c) COX-3
d) COX-4

Answer: B. Inhibiting or blocking COX-1, the good COX, can result in bad things: gastric erosion and ulcers, kidney impairment and bleeding. Suppresssing COX-2, the bad COX, can result in good things like suppressing inflammation, reducing pain and fever, and protecting against colon cancer.

Question M2. Results of blocking COX-2

Drugs like ibuprofen, naproxen, and meloxicam affect cyclooxygenase. When we have inhibition of cyclooxygenase-2 (COX-2) we might expect all of the following except:

a) Analgesia and antipyresis
b) Colorectal cancer protection
c) Gastric ulcers
d) Suppressed inflammation

Question M2. Results of blocking COX-2

Drugs like ibuprofen, naproxen, and meloxicam affect cyclooxygenase. When we have inhibition of cyclooxygenase-2 (COX-2) we might expect all of the following except:

a) Analgesia and antipyresis
b) Colorectal cancer protection
c) Gastric ulcers
d) Suppressed inflammation

Answer: C. Gastric ulcers. A gastric ulcer would likely result from blocking the good COX, COX-1. However, if we block COX-2, the bad COX, we get analgesia (pain reduction), antipyresis (fever reduction), colorectal cancer protection, and suppressed inflammation.

QUESTION M3. IBUPROFEN VS ACETAMINOPHEN

Often patients ask about the difference between ibuprofen and acetaminophen. Acetaminophen and ibuprofen share all of the following therapeutic effects except:

a) Analgesia
b) Antiinflammatory
c) Antipyresis
d) Pain relief

Question M3. Ibuprofen vs acetaminophen

Often patients ask about the difference between ibuprofen and acetaminophen. Acetaminophen and ibuprofen share all of the following therapeutic effects except:

a) Analgesia
b) Antiinflammatory
c) Antipyresis
d) Pain relief

Answer: B. antiinflammatory. While acetaminophen and ibuprofen can provide pain relief (analgesia) and fever reduction (antipyresis), only ibuprofen can provide anti-inflammatory effects. So, we have two basic branches: the drug that can't affect inflammation and the one that can.

QUESTION M4. THE CELECOXIB ADVANTAGE

4) What was thought of as a breakthrough was a selective cyclooxygenase inhibitor that might reduce GI distress from NSAID use. An arthritic patient with a history of GI distress and bleed might be a candidate for:

a) Celecoxib
b) Ibuprofen
c) Naproxen
d) Meloxicam

Question M4. The celecoxib advantage

4) What was thought of as a breakthrough was a selective cyclooxygenase inhibitor that might reduce GI distress from NSAID use. An arthritic patient with a history of GI distress and bleed might be a candidate for:

a) **Celecoxib**
b) Ibuprofen
c) Naproxen
d) Meloxicam

Answer: A. celecoxib. Celecoxib was meant to protect against GI distress, but cardiac issues came up as patients took it, reducing its utilization. Ibuprofen, naproxen, and meloxicam would likely eventually cause GI distress.

QUESTION M5. THE DAILY ASPIRIN ISSUE

In pharmacology, the best practice in using a medication can change even with the most common medicines. What concern about daily aspirin led to a change in the way prescribers look at it for protecting against cardiac events?

a) Bleed risk that can outweigh protective benefit
b) No longer suppresses platelet aggregation
c) No longer protects against MI
d) No longer protects against stroke

Question M5. The daily aspirin issue

In pharmacology, the best practice in using a medication can change even with the most common medicines. What concern about daily aspirin led to a change in the way prescribers look at it for protecting against cardiac events?

    a) Bleed risk that can outweigh protective benefit
    b) No longer suppresses platelet aggregation
    c) No longer protects against MI
    d) No longer protects against stroke

Answer: A. Bleed risk that can outweigh protective benefit. While aspirin still suppresses platelet aggregation and can work to prevent MI and stroke in patients, the bleed risk is a concern. The new guidelines don't apply to those who had a stroke/heart attack, underwent bypass surgery or had a stent procedure. These new guidelines apply to otherwise healthy adults and elderly with a high internal bleed risk.

QUESTION M6. NSAID DOSING INTERVALS

Parents often turn to over-the-counter medicines when their own parents are sick, but aren't always clear as to the best medicine. The OTC NSAID that would most likely suit an adult patient who often forgets to take his or her medicine is:

    a) Ibuprofen
    b) Naproxen
    c) Meloxicam
    d) Celecoxib

Question M6. NSAID dosing intervals

Parents often turn to over-the-counter medicines when their own parents are sick, but aren't always clear as to the best medicine. The OTC NSAID that would most likely suit an adult patient who often forgets to take his or her medicine is:

a) Ibuprofen
b) Naproxen
c) Meloxicam
d) Celecoxib

Answer: B. Naproxen is over-the-counter and lasts up to 8 to 12 hours, so it only needs to be taken a few times a day. Ibuprofen is also over the counter, but a patient might need to take that four times daily. Meloxicam and celecoxib can be taken once or twice daily, respectively, but both require a prescription.

QUESTION M7. ACETAMINOPHEN DOSAGES

7) When a patient asks what dose he or she should take, often there are other factors that change the recommendation. With acetaminophen, we might need to adjust the dose based on the patient having a history of alcoholism.

- a) 1 gram/day
- b) 2 grams/day
- c) 3 grams/day
- d) 4 grams/day

Question M7. Acetaminophen dosages

7) When a patient asks what dose he or she should take, often there are other factors that change the recommendation. With acetaminophen, we might need to adjust the dose based on the patient having a history of alcoholism.

    a) 1 gram/day
    b) 2 grams/day
    c) 3 grams/day
    d) 4 grams/day

Answer: B. 2 grams per day or 2,000 milligrams daily. While the upper limit of safety can go up to 4,000 milligrams per day, a patient who consistently takes in alcohol or who has an overdose of acetaminophen will damage his or her liver.

QUESTION M8. COMBINATION ANALGESICS

8) Sometimes a combination medicine will have a single brand name like Excedrin. Excedrin has three medications; which of the following best describes a medication absent from Excedrin?

a) Abatacept
b) Acetaminophen
c) Acetylsalicylic acid
d) Caffeine

Question M8. Combination analgesics

8) Sometimes a combination medicine will have a single brand name like Excedrin. Excedrin has three medications; which of the following best describes a medication absent from Excedrin?

a) **Abatacept**
b) Acetaminophen
c) Acetylsalicylic acid
d) Caffeine

Answer: A. Abatacept is a disease modifying anti-rheumatic drug, DMARD; each of acetaminophen, aspirin (ASA) and caffeine are in Excedrin.

QUESTION M9. OPIOID RECEPTORS

9) We often use Greek letters to represent receptors in the body. With opioids, the mu and kappa receptors are prominent. We would expect all of the following effects from the kappa receptor except?

    a) Analgesia
    b) Decreased GI motility
    c) Respiratory depression
    d) Sedation

Question M9. Opioid receptors

9) We often use Greek letters to represent receptors in the body. With opioids, the mu and kappa receptors are prominent. We would expect all of the following effects from the kappa receptor except?

a) Analgesia
b) Decreased GI motility
c) **Respiratory depression**
d) Sedation

Answer: C. Respiratory depression falls under the mu receptor as do euphoria and physical dependence. Analgesia, decreased GI motility and sedation, are under the kappa receptor.

QUESTION M10. *DEA Schedules*

The Drug Enforcement Agency, DEA, created drug schedules to provide guidance as to a drug's addiction potential. The DEA schedule II would most likely include which pair of medicines?

a) Heroin and ecstasy
b) Fentanyl and oxycodone
c) Acetaminophen/codeine and testosterone
d) Tramadol and alprazolam

Question M10. DEA Schedules - Drugs

10) The Drug Enforcement Agency, DEA, created drug schedules to provide guidance as to a drug's addiction potential. The DEA schedule II would most likely include which pair of medicines?

a) Heroin and ecstasy
b) Fentanyl and oxycodone
c) Acetaminophen/codeine and testosterone
d) Tramadol and alprazolam

Answer: B. fentanyl and oxycodone fall under DEA schedule II, the most addictive but still legal medication class. Heroin and ecstacy are on DEA schedule I; acetaminophen / codeine and testosterone are included on DEA schedule III; and tramadol and alprazolam are listed on DEA schedule IV.

QUESTION M11. DEA SCHEDULES - TRENDS

11) The Drug Enforcement Agency's drug schedules follow a clear trend. The DEA schedule number _____ as the abuse and dependence potential _____.

    a) Increases; stays the same
    b) Decreases; decreases
    c) Decreases; stays the same
    d) Increases; decreases

Question M11. DEA Schedules - trends

11) The Drug Enforcement Agency's drug schedules follow a clear trend. The DEA schedule number _____ as the abuse and dependence potential _____.

a) Increases, stays the same
b) Decreases, decreases
c) Decreases, stays the same
d) Increases, decreases

Answer: D. Increases, decreases. As we move from DEA Schedule I, the most addictive and illegal medicines to DEA Schedule V, the least addictive, but still controlled substances, the DEA Schedule number increases as the abuse and dependence potential decreases.

QUESTION M12. OPIOID POTENCY

12) Potency between medications can vary significantly, such that if one drug were mistakenly replaced for another, we would have a large disparity in the toxic or therapeutic effect. If we measured the potency of morphine against fentanyl, we would expect that 200 mcg of morphine would be as potent as:

   a) 2 mcg of fentanyl
   b) 4 mcg of fentanyl
   c) 0.02 mcg of fentanyl
   d) 0.04 mcg of fentanyl

Question M12. Opioid potency

12) Potency between medications can vary significantly, such that if one drug were mistakenly replaced for another, we would have a large disparity in the toxic or therapeutic effect. If we measured the potency of morphine against fentanyl, we would expect that 200 mcg of morphine would be as potent as:

a) 2 mcg of fentanyl
b) 4 mcg of fentanyl
c) 0.02 mcg of fentanyl
d) 0.04 mcg of fentanyl

Answer: A. 2 mcg of fentanyl. If the conversion factor is 100 to 1, that is fentanyl is 100 times more potent than morphine, then we could set the problem up this way:

200 mcg morphine x (1 mcg fentanyl/100 mcg morphine)

= 2 mcg of fentanyl

Question M13. Opioid Antagonist

13) Often there are specific side effects that we worry about the most, or that easily come to mind. If we detected opioid toxicity, we would expect to give an opioid antagonist like:

a) Naloxone
b) Meperidine
c) Fentanyl
d) Oxycodone

Question M13. Opioid antagonist

13) Often there are specific side effects that we worry about the most, or that easily come to mind. If we detected opioid toxicity, we would expect to give an opioid antagonist like:

a) **Naloxone**
b) Meperidine
c) Fentanyl
d) Oxycodone

Answer: A. Naloxone (Narcan). The brand name's Narcan or narcotic antagonist gives it away, but if you want to learn 8 opioids quickly, use the first letters of the mnemonic "My my my freaking head hurts ouch ouch," to remember morphine, meperidine, methadone, fentanyl, hydrocodone with acetaminophen, hydrocodone with ibuprofen, oxycodone, and oxycodone with acetaminophen.

QUESTION M14. OPIOID TOXICITY TRIAD

Three issues form the opioid toxicity triad as they relate to overdose. While we would monitor vitals before giving an opioid antagonist, the signs/symptoms of the triad would include all of the following except:

a) Respiratory depression
b) Severe sedation/coma
c) Mydriasis
d) Miosis

Question M14. Opioid toxicity triad

Three issues form the opioid toxicity triad as they relate to overdose. While we would monitor vitals before giving an opioid antagonist, the signs/symptoms of the triad would include all of the following except:

a) Respiratory depression
b) Severe sedation/coma
c) Mydriasis
d) Miosis

Answer: C. Mydriasis. Rather than having wide open pupils, mydriasis, opioid toxicity could result in miosis, pinpoint pupils, respiratory depression, and severe sedation/coma. Note the two dots on top of the two "i" letters in miosis and opioid to remember little pupils.

QUESTION M15. MIGRAINE PATHOLOGY

There are four primary steps in the pathology of a migraine; these include all of the following except:

a) Neural trigger
b) Vasoconstriction
c) Inflammation
d) Neural activation
e) Signal amplification

Question M15. Migraine pathology

There are four primary steps in the pathology of a migraine; these include all of the following except:

a) Neural trigger
b) **Vasoconstriction**
c) Inflammation
d) Neural activation
e) Signal amplification

Answer: B. Vasoconstriction is part of the mechanism of action to help stop a migraine, but vasodilation is what is thought to cause the migraine. Neural trigger, inflammation, neural activation, and signal amplification are each part of the process.

QUESTION M16. ABORTIVE VERSUS PROPHYLACTIC MIGRAINE TREATMENTS

A patient hopes to have fewer migraines. He or she knows that there are medications that can stop a migraine attack and others that can prevent one. Each of the medications below is considered a prophylactic medication except:

a) Sumatriptan
b) Divalproex
c) Amitriptyline
d) Propranolol

Question M16. Abortive versus prophylactic migraine treatments

A patient hopes to have fewer migraines. He or she knows that there are medications that can stop a migraine attack and others that can prevent one. Each of the medications below is considered a prophylactic medication except:

a) **Sumatriptan**
b) Divalproex
c) Amitriptyline
d) Propranolol

Answer: A. Sumatriptan is an abortive migraine medication that would stop an attack. Divalproex (an antiepileptic), amitriptyline (a tricyclic antidepressant), and propranolol (a beta blocker) are all useful for preventing migraines.

QUESTION M17. RECEPTOR NAMING

Often, students confuse agonistic and antagonistic actions, or sub-receptor classes. If someone says he or she is on a triptan for migraines, we expect this to be the mechanism of which action:

a) 5-HT3 antagonist
b) 5-HT3 agonist
c) 5-HT1 antagonist
d) 5-HT1 agonist

Question M17. Receptor naming

Often, students confuse agonistic and antagonistic actions, or sub-receptor classes. If someone says he or she is on a triptan for migraines, we expect this to be the mechanism of which action:

a) 5-HT3 antagonist
b) 5-HT3 agonist
c) 5-HT1 antagonist
d) **5-HT1 agonist**

Answer: D. 5HT1 receptor agonist. The migraine specific triptans are 5 HT 1B/1D receptor agonists. Some confuse these migraine medications with the antiemetic ondandestron's mechanism as a 5-HT3 antagonist.

QUESTION M18. NSAIDS, DMARDS, GLUCOCORTICOIDS

Three primary drug classes to treat rheumatoid arthritis include NSAIDs, DMARDs, and glucocorticoids. All three classes can help relieve symptoms, but only one can delay the progression of the disease. Which of the following medications represents a drug that could delay progression of rheumatoid arthritis?

a) Ibuprofen
b) Meloxicam
c) Prednisone
d) Methotrexate

Question M18. NSAIDS, DMARDS, Glucocorticoids

Three primary drug classes to treat rheumatoid arthritis include NSAIDs, DMARDs, and glucocorticoids. All three classes can help relieve symptoms, but only one can delay the progression of the disease. Which of the following medications represents a drug that could delay progression of rheumatoid arthritis?

a) Ibuprofen
b) Meloxicam
c) Prednisone
d) Methotrexate

Answer: D. Methotrexate is a DMARD; ibuprofen and meloxicam are NSAIDs, and prednisone is a glucocorticoid or steroid for inflammation. Only the DMARD, methotrexate, can delay disease progression.

QUESTION M19. BISPHOSPHONATES KINETICS

Of the four pharmacokinetic principles (absorption, distribution, metabolism and excretion), absorption is critical with bisphosphonates. When giving ibandronate, which of the following instructions would you give a patient?

a) Take without food
b) Take with food
c) It's okay to have coffee, but not food
d) It's okay to have juice, but not food

Question M19. Bisphosphonates kinetics

Of the four pharmacokinetic principles (absorption, distribution, metabolism and excretion), absorption is critical with bisphosphonates. When giving ibandronate, which of the following instructions would you give a patient?

a) **Take without food**
b) Take with food
c) It's okay to have coffee, but not food
d) It's okay to have juice, but not food

Answer: A. Take without food. Even the smallest amount of food can ruin the absorption of bisphosphonates like ibandronate or alendronate. While it may seem okay to drink liquid, in this case, coffee and juice would still affect the absorption.

QUESTION M20. XANTHINE OXIDASE INHIBITORS

Gout is a condition of uric acid buildup, often in the big toe. While some medications can treat the condition in an acute flare-up, which would work to prevent the flare-up by inhibiting xanthine oxidase and uric acid buildup?

a) Ibuprofen
b) Naproxen
c) Febuxostat
d) Aspirin

Question M20. Xanthine oxidase inhibitors

Gout is a condition of uric acid buildup, often in the big toe. While some medications can treat the condition in an acute flare-up, which would work to prevent the flare-up by inhibiting xanthine oxidase and uric acid buildup?

a) Ibuprofen
b) Naproxen
c) Febuxostat
d) Aspirin

Answer: C. Febuxostat is a xanthine oxidase inhibitor that would decrease uric acid. All of the other medications (ibuprofen, naproxen, and aspirin) are NSAIDs that are more appropriate for acute treatment

CHAPTER 3 RESPIRATORY

I. ANTIHISTAMINES AND DECONGESTANTS

We divide **antihistamines** into two generations: first and second. **Diphenhydramine (Benadryl)** is a first-generation antihistamine. In addition to its ability to improve allergy symptoms, it usually makes patients sleepy. The second-generation agents cannot pass through the blood-brain barrier and into the central nervous system, which limits the degree of drowsiness patients experience. This second generation includes **cetirizine (Zyrtec)** and **loratadine (Claritin)**.

My students came up with a useful / helpful / creative visual to remember the difference between histamine-1 and histamine-2 receptors called the antihistamine snowman. They pictured H_1 in the snowman's head because he has only one carrot for his nose, and allergies usually happen in the head / nose. They pictured H_2 as the snowman's belly because that's where gastroesophageal reflux disease (GERD) and hyperacidity happen.

Nasal decongestants like **pseudoephedrine (Sudafed)** constrict blood vessels in the nose and sinuses, reducing the amount of mucus that is formed, and can be found in combination with antihistamines. Usually you will see the brand or generic name followed by a hyphen "D" for decongestant, like **Claritin-D** to indicate that **pseudoephedrine** is a product ingredient. These are not over-the-counter (OTC), but behind the counter (BTC) because you have to show an ID to purchase them.

OTC Antihistamine 1st-generation

Diphenhydramine (Benadryl)
dye-fen-HIGH-dra-mean (BEN-uh-drill)

> Many students on YouTube videos and Quizlet notecards mistake **diphenhydramine's** "i-n-e" as a stem because many antihistamines end in "ine." However, so does **morphine** and roughly 20% of all generic names. There is not really a good stem for antihistamines because of this. You can remember the brand name by recognizing **Benadryl** <u>bene</u>fits you by <u>dry</u>ing up your runny nose. Some students also associated the "B" in **Benadryl** with the BBB, the Blood Brain Barrier, which **Benadryl** can pass through. Manufacturers use **diphenhydramine** as the "P-M" in many sleep aids, so associating the "B" in **Benadryl** with bedtime makes sense.

Hydroxyzine (Atarax)
high-DROCKS-ih-zeen (AT-uh-racks)

> The "x-y-z" inside **hydro<u>xyz</u>ine** matches the brand name of a third-generation antihistamine **Xyzal**.

OTC Antihistamine 2nd-generation

Cetirizine (Zyrtec)
seh-TIE-rah-zine (ZEER-teck)

> Pronounce the "t-i-r" in **cetirizine** as tear, like teardrop, and I think of **cetirizine** protecting me from tearing from eyes affected by allergies.

Loratadine (Claritin)
lore-AT-uh-dean (KLAR-eh-tin)

The "–atadine" stem (used to be "–tadine") is helpful in distinguishing **loratadine** from the "–tidine" stem in the H₂ receptor antagonists **famotidine** and **nizatidine.** The **Claritin** "clear" commercials resonate with the drug's function of clearing one's head from allergies or clear eyes relieved from allergy.

OTC ANTIHISTAMINE 3RD-GENERATION

Fexofenadine (Allegra)
fek-sew-FEH-nuh-deen (uh-LEG-ruh)

The third-generation antihistamine **fexofenadine (Allegra)** is a safe active metabolite of **terfenadine (Seldane),** a drug the manufacturer removed from the market because of cardiac side effects

Levocetirizine (Xyzal)
Lee-vo-sih-TEER-uh-zeen (Zigh-zowl)

The "x-y-z" inside **hydroxyzine** matches the brand name of a third-generation antihistamine **Xyzal**. The Xyzal owl mascot is kind of ironic as owls come out at night, but this is relatively non-sedating. Maybe it's more about being smart like an owl for using Xyzal and it kind of sounds like owl at the end.

OTC ANTIHISTAMINE- EYE DROPS

Olopatadine (Patanol, Pataday)
oh-low-PAH-tuh-deen (PAT-uh-nawl, PAT-uh-day)

From oral antihistamines, I moved to ophthalmic (eye) and nasal forms. **Olopatadine (Patanol,**

131

Pataday) shares the "–atadine" antihistamine stem of **lor<u>atadine</u>**. The two "o's" at the beginning of the generic **<u>o</u>l<u>o</u>patadine** look like eyes.

ANTIHISTAMINE- NASAL SPRAY

Azel<u>astine</u> (Astelin)
ah-ZUH-lah-steen (ASS-tih-Lynn)

> **Azelastine (Astelin)** is a medicine you <u>st</u>ick <u>in</u> your nose. Prescription drugs sometimes transition to over-the-counter (OTC), so I just put **mometasone (Nasonex),** alphabetically before another allergic rhinitis steroid **triamcinolone (Nasacort Allergy 24 HR)**.

OTC ANTIHISTAMINE 2ND-GENERATION / DECONGESTANT

Lor<u>atadine</u> / Pseudoephe<u>drine</u> (Claritin-D)
lore-AT-uh-dean / Sue-doe-uh-FED-rin (KLAR-eh-tin dee)

> Because **pseudoephedrine** has 15 letters, manufacturers abbreviate it as "hyphen D" for decongestant. Therefore, adding **loratadine**, an antihistamine, to **pseudoephedrine** a decongestant, helps with both runny and stuffy noses.

OTC DECONGESTANTS

Pseudoephe<u>drine</u> (Sudafed)
Sue-doe-uh-FED-rin (Sue-duh-FED)

> If you take out the second "e" and drop the "rine" from **pseudoephedrine**, you get the pronunciation

of **Sudafed**. One student said she was p-h-e-d up with being congested and that's how she remembered it.

Phenylephrine (NeoSynephrine)
FEN-ill-EF-rin (KNEE-oh-sin-EF-rin)

> **Phenylephrine** sounds a bit like **pseudoephedrine** – they are both decongestants. Patients recognize **pseudoephedrine** by the "hyphen D" and **phenylephrine** by the "PE" abbreviation. **Phenylephrine** is not as strong as **pseudoephedrine** and that's one reason it's available OTC, while **pseudoephedrine** is not.

Oxymetazoline (Afrin)
ox-EE-meh-taz-oh-lin (AF-rin)

> **Oxymetazoline** takes us from physically behind-the-counter (BTC) oral **pseudoephedrine** to over-the-counter oral **phenylephrine** to the intranasal decongestant **oxymetazoline**. The "**Afrin**" brand name sounds like the "ephrine" that forms the ending of **phenylephrine** so you can relate the two decongestants.

II. ALLERGIC RHINITIS STEROID, ANTITUSSIVES AND EXPECTORANTS

Allergic rhinitis is an inflammation (-itis) of the nose (rhin-). We treat it with a local steroid like **triamcinolone (Nasacort Allergy 24HR)**. Nasal steroids don't work right away like a topical decongestant such as **oxymetazoline (Afrin)** might; rather, it takes weeks of use until a patient feels relief.

Because the name "**Robitussin**" has been associated with cough relief so long, many students mistakenly confuse plain **Robitussin** (just **guaifenesin**) with **Robitussin DM (guaifenesin / dextromethorphan)**. In **Robitussin DM**, the **guaifenesin** acts as an expectorant to lyse (break up) mucous and chest congestion, while the **DM (dextromethorphan)** acts as the antitussive or cough suppressant. In severe cases, a **codeine**-based prescription product such as **guaifenesin / codeine (Cheratussin AC)** may be used.

OTC ALLERGIC RHINITIS STEROID NASAL SPRAY

Fluticasone (Flonase)
flue-TIC-uh-sewn / (flow-NASE)

> Recognize the steroid **fluticasone** by the unofficial "sone." This fluticasone, brand **Flonase** is for allergic rhinitis in the nose with the -nase ending unlike **Flovent** which is for asthma.

Mometasone nasal inhaler (Nasonex)
moh-MEH-tuh-sewn (NAY-zuh-necks)

> Prescription drugs sometimes transition to over-the-counter (OTC), so I just put **mometasone (Nasonex),** alphabetically before another allergic rhinitis steroid **triamcinolone (Nasacort Allergy 24 HR)**.

Triamcinolone (Nasacort Allergy 24HR)
try-am-SIN-oh-lone (NAY-zuh-cort)

> There is no recognized stem in **triamcinolone**, but often "o-n-e," pronounced like I "own" something, matches the "o-n-e" at the end of **testosterone**, a more familiar steroid. The brand name **Nasacort**

reads like a story: "Nasa" for nose, "cort" for corticosteroid, "Allergy" for allergic rhinitis, and "24HR" for how long it works.

OTC Antitussive / Expectorant

**Guaifenesin / Dextromethorphan
(Mucinex DM / Robitussin DM)**
*gwhy-FEN-uh-sin / decks-trow-meth-OR-fan
(MEW-sin-ex dee-em, row-beh-TUSS-in dee-em)*

> **Guaifenesin**, pronounced as if you put a "g" in front of "why," is an expectorant, something that lyses or breaks up mucous. Students remember this because Mr. Mucus from the **Mucinex** commercials is green, which also starts with a "g." **Robitussin** "robs" your cough and "tussin" resembles "tussive." Antitussives are anti-cough medicines.

RX Antitussive / Expectorant

Guaifenesin / Codeine (Cheratussin AC)
gwhy-FEN-uh-sin / CO-dean (CHAIR-uh-tuss-in ay-see)

> Sometimes **dextromethorphan (DM)** isn't enough and the patient needs **codeine** to suppress a cough. Most students know **codeine**, but cough and **codeine** both start with "co" and that seems to help. The "chera" in **Cheratussin** comes from the product's cherry flavoring. Some are not sure what the "AC" means; some students think "anti-cough" al-though it's probably "and codeine."

RX Antitussive

Benzonatate (Tessalon Perles)
BENZ-on-uh-tayte (TESS-uh-lawn PURLZ)

> **Benzonatate (Tessalon Perles)** doesn't work like
> codeine, but as a local anesthetic to decrease the
> sensitivity of lung receptors, reducing your need to
> cough. The "Tess" looks like "<u>tuss</u>ive" and you can
> think of getting a pearl (as from a oyster) stuck in
> your throat. This drug is not in any way an
> anxiolytic (benzodiazepine), but it's interesting that
> the name contains the letters "b-e-n-z-o."

III. ASTHMA

Asthma is a disease of bronchoconstriction (the lung's
branches tighten) and inflammation. For immediate relief
during an attack, an **albuterol (ProAir HFA)** inhaler is the
short-acting bronchodilator that will reverse the
bronchoconstriction. **Proventil** is also a brand name for
nebulized (a form of mist) **albuterol**. Oral steroids such as
methylprednisolone (Medrol) and **prednisone (Deltasone)**
help reduce lung inflammation after a severe attack.

The combination inhalers **fluticasone / salmeterol (Advair)**
or **budesonide / formoterol (Symbicort)** provide relief from
both inflammation and bronchoconstriction by combining a
steroid and long-acting beta$_2$ receptor agonist (which
bronchodilates). Notice that many steroids have "sone" not
an official stem, at the end of their names, and that beta$_2$
receptor agonists have the stem "–terol" in the suffix. These
long-acting combinations prophylactically prevent asthma
attacks.

Ipratropium in **DuoNeb** and **Tiotropium (Spiriva)** are
anticholinergic medications. Often these medications cause
dry mouth, constipation and other unwanted adverse

effects. However, **ipratropium** and **tiotropium (Spiriva)** affect the smooth muscle of the lungs, allowing for bronchodilation and relaxation of the bronchi. Both **albuterol** and **ipratropium** bronchodilate. One is an agonist of beta$_2$ receptors and the other is an antagonist of acetylcholine (ACh).

Montelukast (Singulair) inhibits leukotriene receptors. Leukotrienes cause bronchoconstriction, a process that protects the lungs against foreign contaminants. Drugs in this class end in "–lukast."

Omalizumab (Xolair) is an IgE antagonist and a biologic.

ORAL STEROIDS

Dexamethasone (Decadron)
deck-suh-MEH-thuh-sewn (DECK-uh-drawn)

> **Dexamethasone (Decadron)** is another oral steroid with the -sone ending.

Methylprednisolone (Medrol)
meth-ill-pred-NISS-uh-lone (MED-rol)

> A student connected "pred" and "predator of inflammation" for generic **methylprednisolone**. **Methylprednisolone (Medrol)** comes in a 6-day, 21-pill dose pack that gives patients 6 tablets on the first day, 5 on the 2nd, 4 on the 3rd, 3 on the 4th, 2 on the 5th, and 1 on the 6th. This dosing reminds us to taper steroids to allow the adrenal glands time to resume normal function.

Prednisone (Deltasone)
PRED-ni-sewn (DEALT-uh-sewn)

Most students know **prednisone**, but many steroid compounds have this unofficial "sone" ending. In this case, the "pred-" is the official stem and is in the prefix position. Note, we find this stem in the middle of the drug name in the steroid methyl**pred**nisolone.

OPHTHALMIC STEROID

Lote<u>pred</u>nol ophthalmic (Lotemax)
low-tuh-PRED-nawl (LOW-tuh-macks)

> The ophthalmic preparation **lotepredn<u>ol</u> (Lotemax)** has two o's for eyes and comes after the two "pred" oral steroids, **methylprednisolone** and **prednisone**.

INHALED STEROID/BETA2-RECEPTOR AGONIST LONG-ACTING

Budesonide / Form<u>oterol</u> (Symbicort)
byou-DES-uh-nide / four-MOE-ter-all (SIM-buh-court)

> Similar to **fluticasone / salmeterol, budesonide** has the "sone" syllable in the middle of its name, and is pronounced "sone" even though it's spelled "s-o-n." The "–terol" in **formoterol** indicates a beta2 agonist bronchodilator. You can think of the "S-y-m" in the brand name **Symbicort** as symbiotic, meaning "working with," plus "c-o-r-t" for corticosteroid.

Salm<u>eterol</u> / Fluticasone (Advair)
flue-TIC-uh-sewn / Sal-ME-ter-all (ADD-vair)

> Recognize the steroid **fluticasone** by the unofficial "sone," and the long-acting bronchodilator **salmeterol** by the "-terol" stem. The brand name **Advair** seems like "<u>ad</u>d two drugs to get <u>air</u>."

INHALED STEROID

Budesonide (Rhinocort, Pulmicort Flexhaler)
byou-DES-uh-nide (RIH-no-kort, PULL-muh-kort FLECKS-hailer)

> **Budesonide (Rhinocort, Pulmicort flexhaler)** bears a resemblance to **fluticasone** in that it comes as an over-the-counter nasal spray and prescription inhaler. "Rhino" is for nose and "cort" is for corticosteroid.

Fluticasone (Flovent HFA, Flovent Diskus, Flonase)
flue-TIC-uh-sewn (FLOW-vent)

> The "sone" ending, while not an official stem, is a useful clue that **fluticasone** is a steroid. In the past, inhalers used to feel cold when patients used them because the chlorofluorocarbon (CFC) propellant spray was similar to Freon, the refrigerant used in air conditioning. However, CFCs damage the ozone layer so the new hydrofluoroalkane (HFA) replaces the CFC propellant. The brand name **Flovent HFA** cleverly uses the first two letters of the generic name **fluticasone**, incorporates f-l-o from "airflow" and adds, "vent" to let the patient know this is administered in the mouth. The d-i-s-k-u-s inhaler is a device that looks like a d-i-s-c-u-s (the Frisbee-like thing used in the Olympics) that uses a dry powder for inhalation rather than a propellant and liquid. **Flonase** is the brand name for **fluticasone** administered nasally, and is available OTC.

BETA₂ RECEPTOR AGONIST SHORT-ACTING

Albuterol (ProAir HFA)
Al-BYOU-ter-all (PRO-air aitch-ef-ay)

> The "-terol" stem of **albuterol** indicates it's a beta-2
> adrenergic agonist that causes bronchodilation.
> Note, the "–terol" stem of **albuterol** does not help
> you know if it's long acting or short-acting; that
> distinction has to be memorized. The brand name
> **ProAir HFA** is straightforward with "Pro" as in "I'm
> for it" and "Air" for airway.

Levalbuterol (Xopenex HFA)
Lev-Al-BYOU-ter-all (ZOH-puh-necks)

> **Levalbuterol (Xopenex)** is the enantiomer of
> **albuterol**, so it should work a little bit better. I think
> of "open" and "exhale" when I see the brand name
> **Xopenex**.

BETA₂ RECEPTOR AGONIST / ANTICHOLINERGIC

Albuterol / Ipratropium (DuoNeb)
Al-BYOU-ter-al / Ih-pra-TROPE-e-um (DUE-oh-neb)

> A "-terol" short-acting bronchodilator like **albuterol**
> can combine with a shorter acting anticholinergic
> like **ipratropium** (as compared to longer-acting
> **tiotropium**) in a nebulized form to treat asthma
> symptoms faster. Instructors use **atropine** as the
> prototype drug for the anticholinergics and you can
> see the "-trop-" stem in **atropine, ipratropium**, and
> **tiotropium**. The brand name **DuoNeb** indicates a
> duo of drugs in nebulized form.

Albuterol / Ipratropium (Combivent)
Al-BYOU-ter-al / Ih-pra-TROPE-e-um (KOM-bih-vent)

> DuoNeb and **Combivent** have identical ingredients, but I wanted to make clear **DuoNeb** is a nebulization solution and **Combivent** is a combined inhaler.

Vilanterol / Umeclidinium (Anoro Ellipta)
vih-LAN-ter-al / uh-meh-clih-DIN-ee-um (uh-NOR-oh eh-LIPT-uh)

> The **-clidinium** suffix indicates a muscarinic receptor is involved as a long-acting muscarinic agonist (LAMA). **Vilanterol**, like other beta agonists has the terol, t-e-r-o-l ending. Note, use the letter "v" in vilanterol as this lasts a very long time as a long-acting beta agonist (LAMA). If you look at the actual inhaler casing, it looks like an ellipse, the most famous of which 52-acre park by the White House and north of the National Mall in Washington D.C. The ellipse is supposed to eclipse COPD.

Fluticasone / Vilanterol / Umeclidinium (Trelegy Ellipta)
flue-TIC-uh-sewn / vih-LAN-ter-al / uh-meh-clih-DIN-ee-um (uh-NOR-oh eh-LIPT-uh)

> **Trelegy Ellipta** adds an inhaled steroid for inflammation. Trelegy resembles the word trilogy, having three in a series in a book or movie just as this has three medicines.

ASTHMA / COPD – ANTICHOLINERGIC LONG-ACTING

Tiotropium (Spiriva)
tie-oh-TROW-pee-um (Spur-EE-va)

Tiotropium has the same "-trop-" stem as **ipratropium** and is the long-acting version. As with the "–terols," the beta$_2$ receptor agonists, you have to memorize which anticholinergic is long-acting vs. short-acting. **Spiriva** takes the "spir" from re<u>spir</u>e.

ASTHMA – LEUKOTRIENE RECEPTOR ANTAGONIST

Monte<u>lukast</u> (Singulair)
Mon-tee-LUKE-ast (SING-you-lair)

Leukotrienes form in leukocytes (white blood cells) and cause inflammation. By blocking them, **montelukast** helps with the inflammatory component of asthma. The "-lukast" stem is very similar to leukotriene. The **Singulair** brand name comes from its once daily "single" dosing and the "air" it helps to bring into the asthmatic lungs.

ASTHMA – ANTI-IgE ANTIBODY

Oma<u>liz</u>umab (Xolair)
oh-mah-liz-YOU-mab (ZOHL-air)

Like **infliximab** for ulcerative colitis, **omalizumab** is a biologic. The "inf-" is a prefix that separates it from other similar drugs. The "-li-" stands for immunomodulator (the target), the "-zu-" stands for humanized (the source) and the "–mab" is for mono<u>clonal</u> <u>anti</u>body. There is a black box warning (a severe warning immediately at the beginning of the package insert) for the possibility of anaphylaxis after the first dose and even a year after the onset of treatment. Therefore, health providers inject **omalizumab** where a medicine for treating anaphylaxis is available. The brand name **Xolair** seems like "exhale" and "air."

IV. Anaphylaxis

Anaphylaxis is a special type of allergic overreaction of the body to something like an insect bite or bee sting. **Epinephrine (EpiPen)** quickly reverses the reaction, keeping the airway open.

Epinephrine (EpiPen)
eh-peh-NEF-rin (EP-ee-pen)

> The word **epinephrine** has a Greek origin. "Epi" means "above," and "neph" means "kidney." Above the kidney is the adrenal gland responsible for the body's natural release of **epinephrine**. The Latinized version of **epinephrine** is adrenaline. The "ad" means "above" and "renal" means "kidney." The **EpiPen** brand name comes from the injector device that looks somewhat like a pen.

RESPIRATORY DRUG QUIZ (LEVEL 1)

Classify these drugs by placing the corresponding drug class letter next to each medication. Try to underline the stems before you start and think about the brand name and function of each drug.

1. Albuterol (ProAir)
2. Cetirizine (Zyrtec)
3. Diphenhydramine (Benadryl)
4. Fluticasone/salmeterol (Advair)
5. Guaifenesin/DM (Robitussin DM)
6. Tiotropium (Spiriva)
7. Loratadine (Claritin)
8. Montelukast (Singulair)
9. Pseudoephedrine (Sudafed)
10. Methylprednisolone (Medrol)

Respiratory drug classes:

A. 1st-generation antihistamine
B. 2nd-generation antihistamine
C. Anticholinergic
D. Decongestant
E. Leukotriene receptor antagonist
F. Expectorant/cough suppressant
G. Oral steroid
H. Nasal steroid
I. Short-acting bronchodilator
J. Steroid / long-acting bronchodilator

RESPIRATORY DRUG QUIZ (LEVEL 2)

Classify these drugs by placing the corresponding drug class letter next to each medication. Try to underline the stems before you start and remember the brand name and function of each drug.

1. Budesonide / formoterol
2. Guaifenesin / codeine
3. Triamcinolone
4. Fluticasone / salmeterol
5. Pseudoephedrine
6. Cetirizine
7. Diphenhydramine
8. Albuterol
9. Montelukast
10. Prednisone

Respiratory drug classes:

A. 1st-generation antihistamine
B. 2nd-generation antihistamine
C. Anticholinergic
D. Decongestant
E. Leukotriene receptor antagonist
F. Expectorant / cough suppressant
G. Oral steroid
H. Nasal steroid
I. Short-acting bronchodilator
J. Steroid / long-acting bronchodilator

PRACTICE EXAM PART 3 RESPIRATORY

QUESTION R1. ANTIHISTAMINES FOR SLEEP

We expect patients who want to use antihistamines to sleep need a first-generation antihistamine. Which of the following would be an appropriate therapy for such a patient?

a) Cetirizine
b) Diphenhydramine
c) Fexofenadine
d) Loratadine

Question R1. Antihistamines for sleep

We expect patients who want to use antihistamines to sleep need a first-generation antihistamine. Which of the following would be an appropriate therapy for such a patient?

a) Cetirizine
b) **Diphenhydramine**
c) Fexofenadine
d) Loratadine

Answer: B, Diphenhydramine (Benadryl) is a sedating 1st generation antihistamine. The PM in Tylenol PM represents this medication and its function, to use at night for rest. Cetirizine (Zyrtec), fexofenadine (Allegra), and loratadine (Claritin) are all 2nd generation antihistamines that minimize the drowsiness component.

QUESTION R2. 1ST VS 2ND GENERATION ANTIHISTAMINES

While self-driving cars are becoming a reality, they haven't hit the mainstream yet. A patient who drives for a ride-share company would definitely want to avoid this medication.

a) Cetirizine
b) Diphenhydramine
c) Levocetirizine
d) Loratadine

Question R2. 1st vs 2nd generation antihistamines

While self-driving cars are becoming a reality, they haven't hit the mainstream yet. A patient who drives for a ride-share company would definitely want to avoid this medication.

a) Cetirizine
b) Diphenhydramine
c) Levocetirizine
d) Loratadine

Answer: B, Diphenhydramine. A person who works in a position where he or she needs to stay alert should consider non-sedating 2nd and 3rd generation antihistamines such as cetirizine, levocetirizine, and loratadine.

QUESTION R3. DECONGESTANTS

A patient comes in and says the loratadine he usually uses for his allergies isn't helping his nasal congestion. You expect the medication a person might want to add without a prescription would include:

a) Epinephrine
b) Fexofenadine
c) Phenazopyridine
d) Pseudoephedrine

Question R3. Decongestants vs antihistamines

A patient comes in and says the loratadine he usually uses for his allergies isn't helping his nasal congestion. You expect the medication a person might want to add without a prescription would include:

a) Epinephrine
b) Fexofenadine
c) Phenazopyridine
d) Pseudoephedrine

Answer: D, Pseudoephedrine is a decongestant. Epinephrine is for anaphylaxis, fexofenadine is a 2nd generation antihistamine, and phenazopyridine is a urinary antiseptic to help with the pain of a UTI.

QUESTION R4. DECONGESTANTS

How long a patient needs to be on a medication often dictates the proper therapeutic choice. While you can use _____ for chronic nasal congestion, we would be concerned using ____ for more than a few days because of rebound congestion.

a) Oxymetazoline / pseudoephedrine
b) Pseudoephedrine / loratadine
c) Pseudoephedrine / oxymetazoline
d) Fexofenadine / loratadine

Question R4. Decongestants

How long a patient needs to be on a medication often dictates the proper therapeutic choice. While you can use _____ for chronic nasal congestion, we would be concerned using ____ for more than a few days because of rebound congestion.

a) Oxymetazoline / pseudoephedrine
b) Pseudoephedrine / loratadine
c) **Pseudoephedrine / oxymetazoline**
d) Fexofenadine / loratadine

Answer: C, Pseudoephedrine and oxymetazoline are two decongestants for chronic and acute decongestion, respectfully. Pseudoephedrine is an oral tablet form and oxymetazoline is a nasal spray.

QUESTION R5. STEROIDS VS. ANTIHISTAMINES

It's common for patients who self-treat and buy medicines over-the-counter to have a misunderstanding of how to take their medications properly. Generally, medications for allergic rhinitis provide some relief in the first day or two; however, this medication could take a few weeks to become effective. Which medicine is this?

a) Cetirizine
b) Diphenhydramine
c) Loratadine
d) Triamcinolone

Question R5. Steroids vs. Antihistamines

It's common for patients who self-treat and buy medicines over-the-counter to have a misunderstanding of how to take their medications properly. Generally, medications for allergic rhinitis provide some relief in the first day or two; however, this medication could take a few weeks to become effective. Which medicine is this?

a) Cetirizine
b) Diphenhydramine
c) Loratadine
d) **Triamcinolone**

Answer: D, Triamcinolone is a glucocorticoid (steroid) for allergic rhinitis. These medications are prophylactic and need to be taken daily to work properly. The other three medications, cetirizine, diphenhydramine, and loratadine are antihistamines.

QUESTION R6. ANTITUSSIVES VS EXPECTORANTS

It's common for patients to want a medicine to stop their non-productive dry coughing. Which medication below would *not* help a patient who has this kind of cough?

a) Codeine
b) Dextromethorphan
c) Guaifenesin
d) Hydrocodone

Question R6. Antitussives vs expectorants

It's common for patients to want a medicine to stop their non-productive dry coughing. Which medication below would *not* help a patient who has this kind of cough?

a) Codeine
b) Dextromethorphan
c) **Guaifenesin**
d) Hydrocodone

Answer: C. Guaifenesin is an expectorant, not an antitussive. Codeine, dextromethorphan, and hydrocodone are all antitussives and would stop a cough.

QUESTION R7. BETA-2 AGONIST VS. STEROID

When treating an asthmatic patient, we want to best understand how a combination medication will help him or her improve his or her symptomology. When a prescriber gives a beta-2 agonist like _____ and a steroid like _____ we expect that both the bronchoconstriction and the inflammation will subside.

    a) Albuterol / salmeterol
    b) Fluticasone / salmeterol
    c) Ipratropium / budesonide
    d) Salmeterol / fluticasone

Question R7. Beta-2 agonist vs. Steroid

When treating an asthmatic patient, we want to best understand how a combination medication will help him or her to improve his or her symptomology. When a prescriber gives a beta-2 agonist like _____ and a steroid like _____ we expect that both the bronchoconstriction and the inflammation will subside.

a) Albuterol / salmeterol
b) Fluticasone / salmeterol
c) Ipratropium / budesonide
d) Salmeterol / fluticasone

Answer: D, Salmeterol / fluticasone. Salmeterol ends with -terol, so we know it's a beta-2 agonist. Fluticasone has the -sone in it, so we can be reasonably sure it's a steroid. The albuterol/salmeterol combination would have included two beta-2 agonists. Fluticasone/salmeterol is steroid/beta-2 agonist, and ipratropium/budesonide includes an anticholinergic and steroid.

QUESTION R8. PROPHYLACTIC MEDICINES

We often see a multitude of medications when treating asthma prophylactically. When looking for an oral medication to directly affect leukotrienes, we'd likely turn to:

a) Albuterol
b) Ipratropium
c) Loratadine
d) Montelukast

Question R8. Prophylactic medicines

We often see a multitude of medications when treating asthma prophylactically. When looking for an oral medication to directly affect leukotrienes, we'd likely turn to:

a) Albuterol
b) Ipratropium
c) Loratadine
d) Montelukast

Answer: D, Montelukast is a leukotriene receptor antagonist and you can find many of the letters from leukotriene in the -lukast, l-u-k-a-s-t stem. Albuterol is a beta agonist, ipratropium is an anticholinergic, and loratadine is a 2nd generation antihistamine.

QUESTION R9. SPECIAL ASTHMA DRUGS

Sometimes benefits outweigh the risks. A drug specifically created for allergy-mediated asthma like _____ is generally reserved for more severe cases because of issues with injection site reactions, respiratory infections, or anaphylaxis.

a) Abatacept
b) Infliximab
c) Omalizumab
d) Omeprazole

Question R9. Special asthma drugs

Sometimes benefits outweigh the risks. A drug specifically created for allergy-mediated asthma like _____ is generally reserved for more severe cases because of issues with injection site reactions, respiratory infections, or anaphylaxis.

a) Abatacept
b) Infliximab
c) Omalizumab
d) Omeprazole

Answer: C, Omalizumab is a monoclonal antibody as designated by the -mab, m-a-b ending. While abatacept and infliximab are both biologics, they are not for allergy mediated asthma. Omeprazole is a proton pump inhibitor for excess acid.

QUESTION R10. STEROID DOSAGE FORMS

It's not uncommon for patients to confuse medications for bronchoconstriction with those for inflammation. After a severe asthma exacerbation, a prescriber might use an oral tablet steroid such as _____ to reduce the inflammation associated with the flare-up.

a) Budesonide
b) Fluticasone
c) Oxycodone
d) Prednisone

Question R10. Steroid dosage forms

It's not uncommon for patients to confuse medications for bronchoconstriction with those for inflammation. After a severe asthma exacerbation, a prescriber might use an oral tablet steroid such as _____ to reduce the inflammation associated with the flare-up.

a) Budesonide
b) Fluticasone
c) Oxycodone
d) Prednisone

Answer: D, Prednisone is a steroid for inflammation. The pred-, p-r-e-d- prefix gives it away. The -sone, -s-o-n-e ending is also often in steroids; however, the question asks for an oral dosage form. Budesonide and fluticasone are both steroids, but inhaled or nasal steroids. Oxycodone has the same three-letter ending as prednisone; however, it is an opioid analgesic for pain.

QUESTION R11. INHALED STEROID SIDE EFFECTS

Some side effects are readily preventable. To avoid _____
we can have the patient rinse out his or her mouth with
water after each use of an ICS medicine like _____.

a) *Candidiasis*, fluticasone
b) *Candidiasis*, salmeterol
c) Rapid heart rate, fluticasone
d) Rapid heart rate, salmeterol

Question R11. Inhaled steroid side effects

Some side effects are readily preventable. To avoid _____ we can have the patient rinse out his or her mouth with water after each use of an ICS medicine like _____.

a) *Candidiasis*, **fluticasone**
b) *Candidiasis*, salmeterol
c) Rapid heart rate, fluticasone
d) Rapid heart rate, salmeterol

Answer: A, Candidiasis, fluticasone. Candidiasis, or more commonly "thrush", appears when patients use steroids without washing out their mouths. The ICS, inhaled corticosteroid, is fluticasone. Salmeterol is a beta-2 agonist and that might cause a rapid heart rate.

QUESTION R12. INHALED STEROID SIDE EFFECTS

A patient says that he's been taking his medication as prescribed but has found that he is quite hoarse. You look and see that _____ is a side-effect of ICS.

a) Constipation
b) Diarrhea
c) Dysphonia
d) Tachycardia

Question R12. Inhaled steroid side effects

A patient says that he's been taking his medication as prescribed but has found that he is quite hoarse. You look and see that _____ is a side-effect of ICS.

a) Constipation
b) Diarrhea
c) Dysphonia
d) Tachycardia

Answer: C, Dysphonia literally means bad + sound. Dysphonia and candidiasis are common side effects of inhaled corticosteroids (ICS) if a patient doesn't wash out his or her mouth with water. Constipation, diarrhea, and tachycardia are not side-effects of inhaled steroids.

QUESTION R13. SABA vs LABA

While abbreviations are common in medicine, they can often be confusing to patients. For example, if a prescriber gives a SABA like _____ and a LABA such as _____ in the treatment plan, we'll expect the patient to use:

a) Albuterol, salmeterol
b) Budesonide, formoterol
c) Fluticasone, salmeterol
d) Salmeterol, albuterol

Question R13. SABA vs LABA

While abbreviations are common in medicine, they can often be confusing to patients. For example, if a prescriber gives a SABA like _____ and a LABA such as _____ in the treatment plan, we expect the patient to use:

a) Albuterol, salmeterol
b) Budesonide, formoterol
c) Fluticasone, salmeterol
d) Salmeterol, albuterol

Answer: A, Albuterol/salmeterol. Albuterol is a short-acting Beta-2 agonist, a SABA, while salmeterol is a long-acting beta-2 agonist, a LABA. Expect that the provider will pair salmeterol with a corticosteroid. Budesonide and fluticasone are inhaled corticosteroids. Formoterol is a LABA like salmeterol.

QUESTION R14. BETA AGONISTS VS ANTIMUSCARINICS

When treating asthma in a single combination product, we might use a SABA/SAMA combination. Which of the following represents this medication pairing?

a) Albuterol, ipratropium
b) Albuterol, tiotropium
c) Ipratropium, albuterol
d) Tiotropium, albuterol

Question R14. Beta agonists vs antimuscarinics

When treating asthma in a single combination product, we might use a SABA/SAMA combination. Which of the following represents this medication pairing?

a) **Albuterol, ipratropium**
b) Albuterol, tiotropium
c) Ipratropium, albuterol
d) Tiotropium, albuterol

Answer: A, Albuterol/ipratropium. Albuterol is a short-acting Beta-2 agonist (SABA) and ipratropium is a long-acting muscarinic agonist (SAMA). Tiotropium is a long-acting muscarinic agonist or LAMA.

QUESTION **R15**. **RESCUE INHALERS**

When a patient has a severe asthma attack and is short of breath, we expect to use _____ because it is the most rapid acting of the medicines below.

a) Albuterol
b) Formoterol
c) Ipratropium
d) Salmeterol

Question R15. Rescue inhalers

When a patient has a severe asthma attack and is short of breath, we expect to use _____ because it is the most rapid acting of the medicines below.

 a) **Albuterol**
 b) Formoterol
 c) Ipratropium
 d) Salmeterol

Answer: A, Albuterol is a rescue inhaler meant to immediately open up airways. Formoterol and salmeterol are long-acting bronchodilators not meant for emergent conditions. Ipratropium is an antimuscarinic.

QUESTION R16. ANAPHYLAXIS

After a bee sting, a patient struggles to breathe and reaches for his epinephrine pen. Epinephrine helps this patient because it acts on:

a) Alpha receptors only
b) Beta receptors only
c) Alpha and beta receptors
d) Neither alpha nor beta receptors

Question 16. Anaphylaxis

After a bee sting, a patient struggles to breathe and reaches for his epinephrine pen. Epinephrine helps this patient because it acts on:

a) Alpha receptors only
b) Beta receptors only
c) **Alpha and beta receptors**
d) Neither alpha nor beta receptors

Answer: C, Alpha and beta receptors. Epinephrine can reverse airway constriction by affecting multiple receptors in the body.

QUESTION R17. INHALER TYPES

There are many inhaler types and sometimes another condition that a patient has dictates which inhaler he or she can or cannot use. A type of inhaler which would be the worst choice for someone with severe arthritis would be:

a) Metered-dose
b) Dry powder
c) Respimat
d) Nebulizer

Question R17. Inhaler types

There are many inhaler types and sometimes another condition that a patient has dictates which inhaler he or she can or cannot use. A type of inhaler which would be the worst choice for someone with severe arthritis would be:

a) **Metered-dose**
b) Dry powder
c) Respimat
d) Nebulizer

Answer: A. Metered dose inhalers require significant dexterity to operate and someone with severe arthritis would struggle to coordinate his or her breathing with pushing the tube down. A dry powder inhaler activated by breath or a nebulizer would be a much better choice.

QUESTION R18. STEROIDS AND DIABETES

While steroids can provide excellent prophylaxis against future asthma attacks or reduce inflammation from a burst dose, we must use caution in diabetics because they can cause:

a) Hypoglycemia
b) Hyperglycemia
c) Tachycardia
d) Bradycardia

Question R18. Steroids and diabetes

While steroids can provide excellent prophylaxis against future asthma attacks or reduce inflammation from a burst dose, we must use caution in diabetics because they can cause:

a) Hypoglycemia
b) Hyperglycemia
c) Tachycardia
d) Bradycardia

Answer: B, Hyperglycemia or raised glucose levels is a concern with steroids. The body's own steroids help release glucose into the bloodstream when the fight or flight response activates presuming the body will need more readily available sugar for energy. However, when using steroids as a therapeutic choice, this becomes a concern. Hypoglycemia is a reduction in glucose levels.

QUESTION R19. OMALIZUMAB SIDE EFFECTS

Omalizumab reduces the amount of IgE available in the blood to reduce the amount of mediator complex released and helping a patient with allergy-related asthma. However, it has many potential adverse drug reactions. Which of the following is not one of them?

a) Anaphylaxis
b) Bradycardia
c) Injection site reactions
d) Respiratory infections

Question R19. Omalizumab side effects

Omalizumab reduces the amount of IgE available in the blood to reduce the amount of mediator complex released and helping a patient with allergy-related asthma. However, it has many potential adverse drug reactions. Which of the following is not one of them?

a) Anaphylaxis
b) Bradycardia
c) Injection site reactions
d) Respiratory infections

Answer: B, Bradycardia. Omalizumab can cause injection site reactions, respiratory infections, and anaphylaxis.

QUESTION R20. ASTHMA DELIVERY SYSTEMS

A toddler needs medication for his asthma. Which of the following delivery systems would work best to provide him with the medicine?

a) Metered-dose inhaler
b) Dry powder inhaler
c) Nebulizer
d) Respimat

Question R20. Asthma delivery systems

A toddler needs medication for his asthma. Which of the following delivery systems would work best to provide him with the medicine?

a) Metered-dose inhaler
b) Dry powder inhaler
c) Nebulizer
d) Respimat

Answer: C, Nebulizer. Someone who has neither an ability to control his or her inhalation to the degree a dry powder inhaler would require, or the dexterity and strength to use a metered-dose inhaler, would likely use a nebulizer.

CHAPTER 4 IMMUNE AND INTEGUMENTARY

I. OTC ANTIMICROBIALS

Antimicrobials, meaning "against microbes," can generally be divided into three classes: **antibiotics** (drugs for bacteria), **antifungals** (drugs for mycoses or fungi), and **antivirals** (drugs for viruses). Antibiotic brand names don't give good information about drugs because they derive from generic names. As such, creating linkages between drug classes so you can group similar antibiotics becomes critical. For example, penicillins and cephalosporins, along with **vancomycin**, affect bacterial cell walls. By putting them near each other on this list, you can group them into a larger category based on function.

Antifungals and antivirals, in contrast, have brand names that allude to their therapeutic effect. Most students try to be ultra-efficient and just memorize generic names. Just as you have more information if you know a first and last name, you know more about a drug by memorizing both generic and brand names. This backup information is critical under the stress of exams or clinical practice.

ANTIBIOTIC CREAM

Neomycin / Polymyxin B / Bacitracin (Neosporin)
knee-oh-MY-sin / pall-EE-mix-en / bah-seh-TRACE-in (KNEE-oh-spore-in)

Neomycin is an aminoglycoside that is generally toxic to the kidney (nephrotoxic) and ears (ototoxic) when used systemically. However, patients can safely use topical preparations containing **neomycin** such as over-the-counter **Neosporin**. The brand **Neosporin** takes "N-e-o" from **neomycin**, "p-o" from **polymyxin B**, and "r-i-n" from **bacitracin**." We associate "spores" with fungi, and this helps link **Neosporin** to fungal infections.

Mupirocin (Bactroban) [RX]
myou-PEER-uh-sin (BACK-truh-ban)

> I added the prescription antibiotic, **mupirocin** (**Bactroban**) for impetigo. The Bactroban brand name "bans bacteria" to treat this condition.

ANTIFUNGAL CREAM

Butenafine (Lotrimin Ultra)
BYOU-ten-uh-feen (LOW-treh-min)

> **Butenafine** treats topical fungal infections like ringworm, jock itch, and athlete's foot. Sometimes you will see the Latin names for these conditions: tinea coporis (ringworm), tinea cruris (jock itch), and tinea pedis (athlete's foot) respectively.

Terbinafine (Lamisil)
tehr-BIN-uh-feen (LAH-muh-sill)

> Then I alphabetically listed the antifungal **terbinafine (Lamisil)** after **butenafine (Lotrimin Ultra)** to connect them. But we often see terbinafine for fungus on toenails, and the two t's starting t, terbinafine and t, toenail help me remember. Also, if

you look at terbinafine's spelling, you can also kind of change the name to "toe-will-be-fine" terbinafine.

Clotrimazole / Betametha<u>sone</u> (Lotrisone) [RX]
klow-TRY-muh-zole (LOW-trih-sewn)

By adding **betamethasone**, a steroid, to **clotrimazole**, an OTC antifungal, the combination becomes prescription-only **Lotrisone**.

VACCINATIONS [SOME RX, SOME ANTIBACTERIAL]

Influenza Vaccine (Fluzone, Flumist)
in-FLU-en-zah VACK-seen (FLEW-zone, FLEW-mist)

While some children might need a prescription for the **influenza vaccine**, adults can walk up to the pharmacy counter and get a flu shot at certain pharmacies. Be careful; generic names with "f-l-u," for example, **<u>flu</u>conazole,** an antifungal, and **<u>flu</u>oxetine**, an antidepressant, refer to a fluorine atom in their chemical structure, not to the influenza virus. The "flu" in the vaccine brand names **F<u>lu</u>zone** and **F<u>lu</u>mist** indicates in<u>flu</u>enza, just like **Tami<u>flu</u>,** an oral medication for influenza infection contains the syllable "flu." The nasal vaccine **Flumist** provide an alternative for patients who don't want an injection.

Varicella (Varivax)
vair-uh-SELL-uh (VAIR-uh-vacks)

Note, **Varivax** prevents varicella (chickenpox) and herpes zoster (shingles) respectively. The "vax" in the brand names indicates "vaccine."

Zoster (Zostavax)
ZAH-stihr (ZAH-stuh-vacks)

> Note, **Zostavax** prevents varicella (chickenpox) and herpes <u>zost</u>er (shingles) respectively. Again, the "vax" in the brand names indicates "vaccine."

ANTIVIRAL (ACUTE)

Docosanol (Abreva)
Do-cah-SAN-all (uh-BREE-vah)

> **Docosanol** is a topical antiviral for cold sores caught and treated early. I thought who would pay twenty dollars for a small tube like that? Then I thought of homecoming dances. So, use **docosanol**, so you can go to the ball. **Abreva**, the brand name, hints at therapeutic effect as **docosanol** "<u>abbrev</u>iates" the time a cold sore lasts.

II. ANTIBIOTICS AFFECTING CELL WALLS

Bacteria have cell walls. Human cells don't (although they do have cell membranes). This introduces *selectivity*. If a drug targets a tissue or structure that bacteria have but humans don't, it should be selective for the bacteria and safe for the patient.

Penicillins were one of the first antimicrobial classes discovered. **Penicillin's** mechanism of action is to open a bacterium's cell wall, like popping a bubble, to kill it. This killing action is termed bactericidal. However, sometimes we see resistance to a single antibiotic like **amoxicillin (Amoxil).** For example, a child with an ear infection finishes a course of "the pink stuff" and remains sick. **Amoxicillin/ clavulanate (Augmentin)** adds the compound clavulanate to protect the **amoxicillin** against an enzyme bacteria produce called a beta-lactamase. The enzyme acquired its name from the chemical structure (a beta lactam) that's in all penicillins. This additional component, **clavulanate**, helps **amoxicillin** work in cases where it had previously failed.

Cephalosporins can have cross-sensitivity with penicillins. Patients allergic to one may be allergic to the other, but this is quite rare. We classify cephalosporins into generations. The first-generation drugs, such as **cephalexin (Keflex)**, don't penetrate the cerebrospinal fluid (CSF), have poor gram-negative bacterial coverage (gram-negative bacteria have an extra protective layer and do not take up a gram stain), and are subject to deactivation by beta-lactamase producing bacteria. As we move to third-generation **ceftriaxone (Rocephin)** and fourth-generation **cefepime (Maxipime)**, we get good penetration into the CSF, good gram-negative coverage and the antibiotics cover bacteria resistant to beta-lactam drugs.

Vancomycin (Vancocin) is sometimes the last line of defense against a sometimes-deadly bacterial infection like <u>m</u>ethicillin-<u>r</u>esistant <u>S</u>taphylococcus <u>a</u>ureus (MRSA). To minimize resistance, a special protocol dictates who can and cannot get **vancomycin.** In rare cases, **vancomycin** can cause a hypersensitivity reaction called red man syndrome. **Vancomycin** has special dosing requirements for patient safety and often pharmacists use their expertise to dose it appropriately so that patients receive optimal drug therapy.

ANTIBIOTICS: PENICILLINS

Amox<u>i</u>cillin (Amoxil)
uh-mocks-eh-SILL-in (uh-MOCKS-ill)

Amoxicillin has the "–cillin" stem that indicates its relationship to the penicillin family. The "a-m-o" probably came from the fact that it's an "amino" penicillin. The "-cillin" stem sounds like "cell-in" and can help you remember that **amoxicillin** or, more generally, **penicillins** destroy the cell wall. The brand name **Amoxil** simply removes an "i-c" and "l-i-n" from the generic name.

Penicillin (Veetids)
pen-ih-SILL-en (VEE-tids)

Penicillin follows **amoxicillin** alphabetically with the -cillin stem.

PENICILLIN / BETA-LACTAMASE INHIBITOR

Amoxicillin / Clavulanate (Augmentin)
uh-mocks-eh-SILL-in / clav-you-LAN-ate (awg-MENT-in)

When **amoxicillin** alone doesn't work**, Augmentin** augments **amoxicillin's** defenses against the bacterial beta-lactamase enzyme with **clavulanate**. I think of the "clavicle," the bone in your shoulder, as protective of the upper lung and associate **clavulanate** with that same protective effect.

CEPHALOSPORINS

Cephalexin (Keflex)
sef-uh-LEX-in (KE-flecks)

With cephalosporins, a newer generation has better properties than the last, relative to what the prescriber is treating. Those advantages include better penetration into the cerebrospinal fluid (CSF), better gram- negative coverage, and better resistance to beta-lactamases. You may lose some gram-positive coverage as you move up the spectrum, however. The "ceph-" is an old stem from the first generation. The new stem "cef-" identifies the newer generations. That's how I remember **cephalexin** as being first generation. The brand name **Keflex** takes some letters from **ceph<u>ale</u>xin** to make its name.

Cef<u>ur</u>oxime (Ceftin) [2ⁿᵈ]
seh-FYOUR-awks-eem (SEF-tin)

> **Cefuroxime** is a second-generation cephalosporin.

Cef<u>d</u>inir (Omnicef) [3ʳᵈ]
SEF-dih-near (awm-NIH-sef)

> **Cefdinir** (**Omnicef**) is a third-generation cephalosporin. It was supposed to kill all the bad bacteria and so is named omni-cef for "all."

Cef<u>tr</u>iaxone (Rocephin)
sef-try-AX-own (row-SEF-in)

> In the generic name, **ceftriaxone's** "cef-" indicates it's a cephalosporin. There is a "tri" in the generic name that you can use to remember it's 3ʳᵈ generation. **Rocephin**, the brand name, seems to come from Hoffman-La<u>Ro</u>che's patent. The drug company took the "Ro" from "La<u>Ro</u>che," and the "ceph" and "in" from ce<u>ph</u>alospor<u>in</u> to make **Ro-ceph-in**.

Cef<u>ep</u>ime (Maxipime) [4ᵗʰ]
SEF-eh-peem (MAX-eh-peem)

> **Cefepime** is a fourth-generation cephalosporin. I've remembered it by thinking of four letters "p-i-m-e"

that are in both the brand name **Maxipime** and the generic name **cefepime**. Also, at the time, **Maxipime** was the <u>maxi</u>mum generation, the fourth and highest. However now there is a fifth-generation cephalosporin.

<u>Ce</u>ftaroline (Teflaro) [5th]
Sef-TARE-uh-lean (teh-FLAHR-oh)

> **Ceftaroline** is a fifth-generation cephalosporin and special because it is active against Methicillin-resistant Staphylococcus aureus (MRSA) and community-acquired pneumonia (CAP). I thought of the "flaro, f-l-a-r-o" as a skin "flare, f-l-a-r-e up" as in the skin staph infection it can treat.

GLYCOPEPTIDE

Van<u>co</u>mycin (Vancocin)
van-co-MY-sin (VAN-co-sin)

> **Vancomycin's** "–mycin" stem isn't very useful for finding its therapeutic class. All it really means is that chemists derived **vancomycin** from the *Strepto<u>my</u>ces* bacteria. I remember the function as "**vancomycin** will <u>van</u>quish MRSA." To remember the brand name **Vancocin**, remove the "my" from **vancomycin**.

III. ANTIBIOTICS – PROTEIN SYNTHESIS
INHIBITORS – BACTERIOSTATIC

We name bacteriostatic **tetracyclines** like **doxycycline (Doryx)** and **minocycline (Minocin)** after the four (tetra) member chemical ring (cycline). Tetracyclines and fluoroquinolones both cause photosensitivity and chelation (binding with cations such as the Ca++ in milk or antacids).

We sometimes call **macrolides** "**erythromycins**" after one of the original drugs in the class. Patients take **azithromycin (Zithromax)** as a double dose on the first day and a single dose the following four days. The double dose is a *loading dose*. Once-daily dosing improves patient compliance. Patients take **clarithromycin (Biaxin)** twice a day – notice the "bi" prefix in the brand name, and we dose **erythromycin (E-Mycin)** four times a day.

Dentists use **clindamycin (Cleocin)** for dental prophylaxis when a patient is penicillin allergic. Patients use it topically for severe acne. When used orally, it can cause a severe condition known as pseudomembranous colitis, also known as antibiotic-associated diarrhea (AAD).

Linezolid (Zyvox) is an oxazolidinone antibiotic that can work on both **methicillin**-resistant *Staphylococcus aureus* (MRSA) and **vancomycin**-resistant enterococci (VRE).

TETRACYCLINES

Doxycycline (Doryx)
docks-ee-SIGH-clean (DOOR-icks).

> I use the "d" in **doxycycline** to remind me that dentists use it to treat periodontal disease. **Doryx**, the brand name, takes the first four letters of **doxycycline** and adds an "r."

Minocycline (Minocin)
MIN-oh-SIGH-clean (MIN-oh-sin)

> **Minocycline**, like **doxycycline** has the **tetracycline** class "-cycline" stem. To create the brand name

Minocin, the manufacturer dropped the "c-y-c-l" and last "e."

Tetracycline (Sumycin)
teh-truh-SIGH-clean (SUE-my-sin)

Tetracycline (Sumycin), although it's essentially unavailable by itself, would follow alphabetically after **doxycycline** and **minocycline**. We see it in *Helicobacter pylori* regimens.

QUAD PEPTIC ULCER DISEASE THERAPIES - BED-MIDNIGHT or MACE

A more comprehensive acrostic mnemonic for the peptic ulcer therapy from my *Memorizing Pharmacology Mnemonics* book might be good to talk about here. The idea is that to treat *Helicobacter pylori* you want to avoid resistance, so you use three antibiotics instead of one or two in addition to an acid reducer. So, two treatment options might look like this:

I use *BED-M, B-E-D-M* (think: "acid in bed at midnight") and MACE, M-A-C-E a weapon, crushing *H. Pylori*.

B, bismuth, has antibiotic properties. Bismuth can have adverse side effects, such as Reye's syndrome, a neurologic condition. Also, watch for salicylism, and tarry black stools and black tongue. The black stools may mimic symptoms of GI bleed, so that's a counseling consideration.

E, esomeprazole, is a proton pump inhibitor to reduce acid.

D, doxycycline, a tetracycline antibiotic. Like using esomeprazole as representative for any PPI, we can substitute other tetracyclines. Doxycycline is a tetracycline we avoid with children to prevent tooth discoloration. Watch also for chelation and sun sensitivity.

M, metro<u>nidazole</u>, an antiprotozoal that can cause metallic taste and nausea. If a patient adds alcohol, this causes a disulfiram reaction that may result in severe vomiting.

The MACE mnemonic reorders drugs from this chapter and an acid reducer.

M, metro<u>nidazole</u>
A, amox<u>icillin</u>
C, clari<u>thromycin</u>
E, esome<u>prazole</u>

MACROLIDES

Az<u>ithromycin</u> (Zithromax Z-Pak)
ay-zith-row-MY-sin" (ZITH-row-max)

> To recognize the three macrolides, **azithromycin,**
> **clarithromycin,** and **erythromycin,** you will see the
> "–mycin" ending, but also a possible infix of "thro-."
> Be careful: there are macrolides without this infix
> and stem. The brand name **Zithromax** takes seven
> letters from **az<u>ithromy</u>cin** to construct its name. The
> **Zithromax Z-pak** is a convenient six-tablet package
> that includes a five-day course, two tablets for a
> loading dose on day one and one tablet for each
> thereafter.

Clari<u>thromycin</u> (Biaxin)
Claire-ITH-row-my-sin (bi-AX-in)

> Gastroenterologists prescribe **clarithromycin** for
> peptic ulcer disease (PUD) triple therapy along with
> **amoxicillin** and a proton pump inhibitor like
> **omeprazole.** The **Biaxin** brand name indicates the

twice daily dosing from the Latin abbreviation b.i.d. or *bis in die.*

Erythromycin (E-Mycin)
err-ith-row-MY-sin (E-MY-sin)

> Some **erythromycin** tablets are bright red and that might be where it got its name. An erythrocyte is a red blood cell, and the word comes from connecting "erythro," the Greek for "red," and "cyte," for cell. The brand name **E-mycin** comes from taking the "rythro" out of the generic name **erythromycin**.

Fidaxomicin (Dificid)
fih-DAKS-oh-my-sin (DIH-fih-sid)

> The "dax" in the name **fidaxomicin (Dificid)** might come from its source, *Dactylosporangium aurantiacum*. The brand name **Dificid** indicates its primary therapeutic use against *Clostridium difficile*.

LINCOSAMIDE

Clindamycin (Cleocin)
clin-duh-MY-sin (KLEE-oh-sin)

> Most students remember the adverse effect CDAD (*Clostridium difficile*-Associated Disease) because there is a "c" and a "da" right after in the generic **clindamycin**. To make the brand name **Cleocin,** the manufacturer replaced the "i-n-d-a-m-y" in **clindamycin** with "e-o."

OXAZOLIDINONE

Linezolid (Zyvox)

LYNN-ez-oh-lid (ZIE-vocks)

> The "-zolid" stem in **linezolid** comes from the
> **oxazolidinone** class. I think it's more helpful to
> think, "Man, **Zyvox** is zolid (solid); it treats two very
> difficult to treat organisms, MRSA and VRE.

IV. ANTIBIOTICS – PROTEIN SYNTHESIS
INHIBITORS – BACTERICIDAL

Bactericidal **aminoglycosides** can damage the kidneys
(nephrotoxicity) and ears (ototoxicity). I think of the "side"
in **aminoglycoside** and "cide" as in "cidal" to remind me
these are killers.

AMINOGLYCOSIDES

Amikacin (Amikin)
am-eh-KAY-sin (AM-eh-kin)

> Some internet sources say that a "cin" ending means
> an aminoglycoside, but that's not necessarily true.
> Many antibiotics end in "c-i-n," so I think it's more
> useful to look at the "a-m-i" that is in the words
> **aminoglycoside**, **amikacin** and **Amikin**. The brand
> name **Amikin** is simply **amikacin** without the "a-c."

Gentamicin (Garamycin)
Jenn-ta-MY-sin (gare-uh-MY-sin)

> Just as practitioners abbreviate **vancomycin** as
> "vanc" in conversation, they abbreviate **gentamicin**
> as "gent." The brand name **Garamycin** is similar to
> **gentamicin** spelled with "**-mycin**" not "**-micin.**"

V. ANTIBIOTICS FOR URINARY TRACT INFECTIONS (UTIS) AND PEPTIC ULCER DISEASE (PUD)

Sulfamethoxazole / trimethoprim (Bactrim) is a combination therapy that affects the folic acid in bacteria. Humans can safely ingest folic acid, so it doesn't affect us adversely. However, sulfa medications can sometimes cause allergic reactions. **Sulfamethoxazole** can even cause a rare but life-threatening condition of the skin and mucous membranes known as Stevens-Johnson syndrome. Sulfa drugs clear urinary tract infections (UTIs) and provide prophylaxis (prevention) of certain infections that commonly occur in immunocompromised patients such as HIV patients.

We sometimes call **fluoroquinolones** "floxacins" after their infix "-fl-" + suffix "-oxacin." Like tetracyclines, fluoroquinolones cause photosensitivity (an increased sensitivity to burning from sunlight) and chelation (a binding with cations such as the Ca++ in milk or antacids). **Fluoroquinolones** have a very unusual side effect in that sometimes they can cause tendon rupture, although rarely.

Metronidazole (Flagyl) treats various infections, including *H. Pylori*, as part of triple therapy. A notable side effect of **metronidazole** is the disulfiram reaction where a patient may experience serious nausea and vomiting. Projectile vomiting is rare, but a vivid way to remember **metronidazole's** adverse effect with alcohol.

OTC URINARY TRACT ANALGESIC

Phenazopyridine (Uristat)
feh-nah-zoe-PY-rih-dean (YOUR-ih-stat)

Phenazopyridine (Uristat) is an over-the-counter urinary tract analgesic that allows a patient to get some relief before she can see her physician for treatment of a bladder infection.

NITROFURAN

Nitrofurantoin (Macrobid, Macrodantin)
nigh-trow-FYOUR-an-toe-in (MAK-row-bid, MAK-row-dan-tin)

Nitrofurantoin (Macrobid, Macrodantin) is a nitrofuran antibiotic, as the first brand name implies, and is taken twice daily as indicated by the "b-i-d" in the name.

Fosfomycin (Monurol)
FAWS-foh-my-sin (mawn-YOUR-all)

The Mon, M-o-n in **Monurol** refers to mono, m-o-n-o meaning it is given in one dose. If the UTI is complicated you might see a single dose every two or three days depending on severity.

DIHYDROFOLATE REDUCTASE INHIBITORS

Sulfamethoxazole / Trimethoprim (SMZ-TMP)
sull-fa-meth-OX-uh-zol e /try-METH-oh-prim
(ess-em-zee / tee-em-pee)

SMZ / TMP is the acronym for **sulfamethoxazole / trimethoprim**. I want to caution you about seeing sulfa in the name and allergic reactions. While sulfa drugs have "s-u-l-f-a" in them, some drugs have sulfa groups in the chemicals structure, but not in the generic name, e.g., **furosemide.** The academic literature doesn't support cross-sensitivity between allergies to sulfa antibiotics and other sulfonamide containing drugs like **furosemide**. The brand name **Bactrim** contains "b-a-c-t-r-i-m" from "<u>bact</u>e<u>rium</u>."

FLUOROQUINOLONES

Ciprof<u>loxacin</u> (Cipro)
sip-row-FLOCKS-uh-sin (SIP-row)

The **quinolone** stem is "-oxacin," but **fluoroquinolones** have the "-fl-" infix also. One student remembered quinolones are for UTIs because Dr. Quinn, Medicine Woman, is female. Women get proportionally more UTIs than men do. By cutting the "–floxacin" stem from the generic name **ciprofloxacin**, the manufacturer made the brand name, **Cipro**.

Gati<u>floxacin</u> ophthalmic (Zymar)
Gah-tih-FLOCKS-uh-sin (ZEYE-mar)

Gatifloxacin ophthalmic (Zymar) is a fluoroquinolone ophthalmic preparation.

Levo<u>floxacin</u> (Levaquin)
Lee-vo-FLOCKS-uh-sin (LEV-uh-Quinn)

Levofloxacin is the left-handed (levo) isomer of **ofloxacin**, another **fluoroquinolone**. The brand name combines the "lev" from <u>lev</u>ofloxacin and "quin" from fluoro<u>quin</u>olone to form **Levaquin**.

Moxi<u>floxacin</u> (Avelox) / [Ophthalmic is **Vigamox**]
Mawks-ee-FLOCKS-uh-sin (AH-vih-locks, VI-guh-mawks)

Moxifloxacin (Avelox, Vigamox). Vigamox is an ophthalmic preparation and contains "v-i" for v̲ision. I don't like seeing the "amox, a-m-o-x" because it makes it look like another type of antibiotic.

Metro̲nidazole (Flagyl)
met-ruh-NYE-duh-zole (FLADGE-ill)

> The generic name **metronidazole** contains one of the three "i's" from nitroimidazole, its parent class. Gastroenterologists use **metronidazole** for peptic ulcer disease (PUD). Note that **metronidazole** is technically an antiprotozoal and students look at the "azole" ending, which is a little similar to "ozoal" from "protozoal." A student learned to give "Flag,"a shorter form of **Flagyl**, for *B. frag* a shortening of the *Bacteroides fragilis* infections.

VI. ANTI-TUBERCULOSIS AGENTS

Prescribers use anti-tuberculosis agents for an extended period (several months) because tuberculosis organisms grow slowly. Multiple drug therapy helps prevent resistance. I use the acronym "r-i-p-e," to remember the four major antituberculosis agents: **r̲ifampin, i̲soniazid, p̲yrazinamide**, and **e̲thambutol**. Non-drug resistant, non-HIV patients take all four drugs for two months, and then **isoniazid** and **rifampin** together for four more months.

R̲ifampin (R̲ifadin)
rif-AM-pin (rif-UH-din)

Students remember that **rifampin** turns secretions like tears, sweat, and urine red with its first letter "r." The brand name **Rifadin** simply replaces the "m-p" from **rifampin** with a "d."

Isoniazid (INH)
eye-sew-NIGH-uh-zid (EYE-en-aitch)

There is no "H" in **isoniazid**, so **INH** comes from the chemical name **iso**n**i**cotinyl**h**ydrazide. The "n-i" in **iso**n**i**azid reminds students that peripheral **n**eur**i**tis is an adverse effect.

Pyrazinamide (PZA)
pier-uh-ZIN-uh-mide (pee-zee-ay)

The "p" in **pyrazinamide** reminds students that an adverse effect is polyarthritis. **Pyra**z**ina**mide's abbreviation is **PZA**.

Ethambutol (Myambutol)
eh-THAM-byou-tall (my-AM-byou-tall)

The "e" for "eyes" or "o" in **ethambut**o**l** helps remind students that optic neuritis is an adverse effect. To make the brand name, the manufacturer replaced the "eth" in **ethambutol** with "my" in **Myambutol** because *My*cobacterium tuberculosis is the causative agent.

VII. Antifungals

Scientists divide antifungals into two general types: systemic (in the body) and dermatologic or topical (on the skin). Before the advent of antifungals, most systemic fungal infections were deadly. **Amphotericin B (Fungizone)** can treat systemic infections. **Fluconazole (Diflucan)** orally treats vaginal yeast infections. **Nystatin (Mycostatin)** can eliminate thrush or yeast infections.

Amphotericin B (Fungizone)
am-foe-TER-uh-sin bee (FUN-gah-zone)

> What about **amphotericin A**? Well, it didn't do anything, so they came up with **amphotericin B**. While the antibacterials' brand names didn't do a very good job helping to indicate their therapeutic effects, this antifungal's brand name, **Fungizone**, makes it easier to know its therapeutic use.

Fluconazole (Diflucan)
flue-CON-uh-zole (die-FLUE-can)

> The "–conazole" ending helps identify **fluconazole** as an antifungal drug. Again, be careful of the "f-l-u" in **fluconazole**, which is for a fluorine atom it contains, not influenza. One student came up with using the first three letters of the brand name **Diflucan** as "Die fungi!"

Ketoconazole (Nizoral)
KEY-tuh-CON-uh-zole (nih-ZUH-rowl)

> The antifungal **ketoconazole (Nizoral)** fits alphabetically with the other "azole" antifungal **fluconazole (Diflucan)**.

Nystatin (Mycostatin)
NIGH-stat-in (MY-co-stat-in)

> **Nystatin** is an interesting generic name because it ends in "statin." A class of cholesterol lowering drugs, the HMG-CoA reductase inhibitors, commonly referred to as "statins," have a similar ending. A better infix + suffix stem for HMG-CoA reductase inhibitors is "vastatin." To keep from thinking **nystatin** was ever a cholesterol lowering "statin," one student remembered the dosage forms nystatin comes in: powder and liquid to swish / spit / swallow. **Mycostatin**, the brand name, dropped the "ny" from **nystatin** and added "Myco," a prefix often seen with <u>myco</u>ses (fungal infections).

VIII. ANTIVIRALS – NON-HIV

Many antivirals have "-vir-" in the middle or at the end of the generic and / or brand name. Drugs for influenza, such as **oseltamivir (Tamiflu)** and **zanamivir (Relenza)** work when taken within 48 hours of the infection. Drugs for herpes infections such as **acyclovir (Zovirax)** and **valacyclovir (Valtrex)** can help prevent recurrences and treat an infection, but they do not cure the disease.

Respiratory syncytial virus (RSV) is usually unproblematic in healthy adults, but in infants younger than one year old, it can be deadly. A drug like the vaccine **palivizumab (Synagis)** can prevent RSV in at-risk patient populations.

INFLUENZA A AND B

Oseltamivir (Tamiflu)
owe-sell-TAM-eh-veer (TA-mi-flue)

Often family members will all get prescriptions for **oseltamivir** if one person is sick enough or if a family member is immunocompromised. The brand name **Tamiflu** alludes to a drug that "tames the flu." It's prescribed for acute influenza or prophylaxis.

Zanamivir (Relenza)
za-NAH-mi-veer (rah-LEN-zuh)

Zanamivir comes in a Diskhaler, a way to get powder to the lungs. The Diskhaler is difficult for patients with dexterity issues, but provides an alternative to **oseltamivir (Tamiflu)**. Think: **Relenza** "**re**presses influ**enza**" virus or **Relenza** makes "influ**enza rel**ent" (give up).

HERPES SIMPLEX VIRUS & VARICELLA-ZOSTER VIRUS (HSV/VSV)

Acyclovir (Zovirax)
ay-SIGH-clo-veer (zo-VIE-racks)

Zovirax treats Varicella-Zoster virus (VSV) and herpes simplex virus (HSV). You can think of **Zovirax** as a drug that axes Zoster virus. Dosing is five times daily.

Valacyclovir (Valtrex)
Val-uh-SIGH-clo-veer (VAL-trex)

Valacyclovir has **acyclovir** in the name because it's the valine ester. A prodrug like **valacyclovir** turns into an active drug in the body, in this case, **acyclovir**. **Valacyclovir** allows for twice daily dosing, so prescribers prefer the oral form of **valacyclovir** to **acyclovir** for patient compliance. The brand name, **Valtrex,** includes the "val" from <u>val</u>acyclovir plus T-rex, and wrecks a virus.

RESPIRATORY SYNCYTIAL VIRUS (RSV)

Pali<u>viz</u>umab (Synagis)
pal-eh-viz-YOU-mab (SIN-uh-giss)

> The prefix "p-a-l-i" has "P" and "I" in it. You can remember **palivizumab** is for pediatrics or infants at risk for RSV. In **palivizumab**, the "pali" is a prefix that separates it from other drugs. The "-vi-" stands for antiviral (the target), the "-zu-" stands for humanized (the source), and the "–mab" is for <u>m</u>onoclonal <u>anti</u>body. This biologic stem + infixes resemble **infliximab (Remicade)** for ulcerative colitis or **omalizumab (Xolair)** for asthma, but with a different clinical purpose.

HEPATITIS

Ente<u>cavir</u> (Baraclude)
en-TEK-uh-veer (BEAR-uh-klewd)

> **Entecavir (Baraclude)** is for active hepatitis infections.

Hepatitis A (Havrix)
heh-puh-TIE-tuss A (HAV-Ricks)

> **Hepatitis A (Havrix)** vaccines are preventative.

Hepatitis B (Recombivax HB)
heh-puh-TIE-tuss B (rih-COM-buh-vacks)

Hepatitis B (Recombivax HB) vaccines are preventative.

HPV

Human papillomavirus (Gardasil)
HYOU-muhn-pah-pih-LOW-muh VI-Russ (GAR-duh-sill)

> **Gardasil** <u>guard</u>s against human papillomavirus (HPV).

IX. ANTIVIRALS – HIV

HIV drugs affect specific targets in the cell or retrovirus. HIV medications, like tuberculosis medications, often work best in drug combinations. I've organized the five HIV drug classes in the order an HIV virus attacks a healthy cell. First, the HIV virus tries to fuse with the cell, then it uses cellular chemokine receptor five (CCR5) to enter the cell. Inside the cell, the HIV virus uses reverse transcriptase, integrase, and protease. HIV medications have three letter abbreviations, as these drugs are not only hard to pronounce, but conversation filled with several multisyllable words can make comprehension difficult.

FUSION INHIBITOR

Enfu<u>vir</u>tide (Fuzeon) (T-20)
En-FYOO-veer-tide (FYOO-zee-on)

> It's easier to remember **enfuvirtide's** brand name **Fuzeon** first because it's a <u>fusion</u> inhibitor. Inside the generic name, you see "vir" for antiviral and we pronounce the "f-u" as FYOO. Put that together and you can remember **enfuvirtide** is **Fuzeon**, a fusion

inhibitor. I use the "T" in "**T-20**" to remember that "tide" is the last syllable in the generic name.

CELLULAR CHEMOKINE RECEPTOR (CCR5) ANTAGONIST

Maraviroc (Selzentry) (MVC)
MARE-uh-VIR-ock (SELLS-en-tree)

> The stem "-vir-" is inside the generic name **maraviroc**. The sub-stem "-viroc" has five letters, with the "c" at the end of the generic name, so you can remember it's a CCR5 antagonist. You can think of **maraviroc** as a "rock" guarding against viral entry. The brand name **Selzentry** sounds a lot like "sentry," someone who guards.

NON-NUCLEOSIDE REVERSE TRANSCRIPTASE INHIBITORS (NNRTIs) WITH 2 NUCLEOSIDE / NUCLEOTIDE REVERSE TRANSCRIPTASE INHIBITORS (NRTIs)

Efavirenz (Sustiva) [NNRTI]
eh-fah-VUH-rihnz (suh-STEVE-uh)

> **Efavirenz (Sustiva)** is an NNRTI. It's brand name indicates it will help sustain the patient as they battle this disease.

Emtricitabine / Tenofovir (Truvada) [NRTIs]
em-truh-SIGH-tuh-bean / tuh-NO-fuh-veer (true-VAH-duh)

> Both **emtricitabine** and **tenofovir (Truvada)** are nucleotide reverse transcriptase inhibitors (NRTIs).

Efavirenz / Emtricitabine / Tenofovir (Atripla) (EFV / FTC / TDF)

eh-FAH-vir-enz / EM-try-SIGH-tah-been / ten-OFF-oh-vir
(ay-TRIP-lah)

> First look at the antiviral sub-class with the stems "-virenz," "-citabine," and "-vir." Then add the other two or three syllables to memorize the whole names of **efavirenz, emtricitabine**, and **tenofovir**. The brand name **Atripla** can be thought of as three drugs, "triple" surrounded by two A's that can stand for "against AIDS."

INTEGRASE STRAND TRANSFER INHIBITOR

Raltegravir (Isentress) (RAL)
ral-TEG-ra-veer (EYE-sen-tress)

> **Raltegravir** is an integrase strand transfer inhibitor. Inside the generic name, you can find the stem "-tegravir" made up of "tegra," a part of integrase and "vir" for antiviral. The brand name **Isentress** also looks like sentry, except it has the "I" to remind you of integrase.

PROTEASE INHIBITOR

Atazanavir (Reyataz) (ATV)
at-uh-ZAN-uh-veer (RAY-uh-taz)

> The protease inhibitor **atazanavir (Reyataz)** fits in alphabetically and has the navir, n-a-v-i-r substem.

Darunavir (Prezista) (DRV)
dar-YOU-nah-veer (Pre-ZIST-uh)

The brand name, in this case, is a little easier. **Prezista** sounds like resist spelled "r-e-z-i-s-t," and the first two letters "p-r" of "protease."

X. MISCELLANEOUS

Albendazole (Albenza) [Anthelmintic]
Al-BEN-duh-zole (Al-BENZ-uh)

> **Albendazole (Albenza)** is an anthelmintic, which means "against worms;"

Hydroxychloroquine (Plaquenil) [Antimalarial]
high-drock-see-KLORE-uh-kwin (PLAH-kwih-nil)

> **Hydroxychloroquine (Plaquenil)** is an antimalarial that was made famous during the pandemic and also has use against rheumatoid arthritis.

Nitazoxanide (Alinia) [Antiprotozoal]
Nigh-tuh-ZOCKS-uh-nyde (Uh-LYNN-ee-uh)
> **Nitazoxanide (Alinia)** is an antiprotozoal.

Immune drug quiz (Level 1)

Classify these drugs by placing the corresponding drug class letter next to each medication. Try to underline the stems before you start and think about the brand name and function of each drug.

1. Amoxicillin (Amoxil)
2. Azithromycin (Zithromax)
3. Cefepime (Maxipime)
4. Ceftriaxone (Rocephin)
5. Fluconazole (Diflucan)
6. Gentamicin (Garamycin)
7. Isoniazid (INH)
8. Levofloxacin (Levaquin)
9. Nystatin (Mycostatin)
10. Valacyclovir (Valtrex)

Immune drug classes:

A. 1st-generation cephalosporin
B. 2nd-generation cephalosporin
C. 3rd-generation cephalosporin
D. 4th-generation cephalosporin
E. Antibiotic: aminoglycoside
F. Antibiotic: fluoroquinolone
G. Antibiotic: macrolide
H. Antibiotic: penicillin
I. Antibiotic: sulfa
J. Antibiotic: tetracycline
K. Anti-fungal
L. Anti-tuberculosis
M. Anti-viral (herpes)
N. Anti-viral (HIV)
O. Anti-viral (influenza)

IMMUNE DRUG QUIZ (LEVEL 2)

Classify these drugs by placing the corresponding drug class letter next to each medication. Try to underline the stems and remember the brand name and drug function.

1. Rifampin
2. Amphotericin B
3. Amikacin
4. Ciprofloxacin
5. Pyrazinamide
6. Acyclovir
7. Cephalexin
8. Sulfamethoxazole / Trimethoprim
9. Erythromycin
10. Oseltamivir

Immune drug classes:

A. 1st-generation cephalosporin
B. 2nd-generation cephalosporin
C. 3rd-generation cephalosporin
D. 4th-generation cephalosporin
E. Antibiotic: aminoglycoside
F. Antibiotic: fluoroquinolone
G. Antibiotic: macrolide
H. Antibiotic: penicillin
I. Antibiotic: sulfa
J. Antibiotic: tetracycline
K. Anti-fungal
L. Anti-tuberculosis
M. Anti-viral (herpes)
N. Anti-viral (HIV)
O. Anti-viral (influenza)

PRACTICE EXAM PART 4
IMMUNE AND INTEGUMENTARY

QUESTION I1: CELL WALL INHIBITORS

While humans and bacteria might have cell membranes, humans lack a cell wall. This allows us to selectively target the bacteria but not the human cell by using a medication like:

a) Cefepime
b) Ciprofloxacin
c) Clarithromycin
d) Clindamycin

Question 11: Cell Wall Inhibitors

While humans and bacteria might have cell membranes, humans lack a cell wall. This allows us to selectively target the bacteria but not the human cell by using a medication like:

a) **Cefepime**
b) Ciprofloxacin
c) Clarithromycin
d) Clindamycin

Answer: A. Cefepime is an example of a cephalosporin medication with the cef, c-e-f prefix. Cephalosporins, like penicillins, act by inhibiting cell-wall synthesis. This leads to bacterial lysis and cell death. Ciprofloxacin is a fluoroquinolone antibiotic which has the -floxacin stem. Clarithromycin is a macrolide antibiotic that has the -thromycin stem. Clindamycin is a lincosamide antibiotic.

QUESTION I2: BACTERIOSTATIC VS. BACTERICIDAL

Some medications kill bacteria and others prevent them from replicating or growing. We expect that ____ would fall under those drugs that only prevent the growth of the bacteria.

a) Amoxicillin
b) Cephalexin
c) Minocycline
d) Vancomycin

Question 12: Bacteriostatic vs. Bactericidal

Some medications kill bacteria and others prevent them from replicating or growing. We expect that ____ would fall under those drugs that only prevent the growth of the bacteria.

 a) Amoxicillin
 b) Cephalexin
 c) Minocycline
 d) Vancomycin

Answer: C. Minocyline. Tetracyclines such as minocycline are bacteriostatic and inhibit bacterial protein synthesis. Penicillins such as amoxicillin, cephalosporins such as cephalexin, and glycopeptides like vancomycin are all bactericidal, meaning that they kill the bacteria outright. All three classes affect the cell wall.

QUESTION 13: ANTIMETABOLITES

An important metabolic product of bacteria is folic acid. Antibiotics that disrupt this pathway can still be selective and cause relatively little harm to humans because we can ingest external folic acid in foods or as a supplement. Which medication would most likely work this way?

a) Aripiprazole
b) Esomeprazole
c) Fluconazole
d) Sulfamethoxazole

Question 13: Antimetabolites

An important metabolic product of bacteria is folic acid. Antibiotics that disrupt this pathway can still be selective and cause relatively little harm to humans because we can ingest external folic acid in foods or as a supplement. Which medication would most likely work this way?

  a) Aripiprazole
  b) Esomeprazole
  c) Fluconazole
  d) Sulfamethoxazole

Answer: D. Sulfamethoxazole takes the place of PABA in the folate synthesis pathway disrupting it. Bacteria have to make their own folate to make DNA, RNA, and proteins so the sulfamethoxazole harms them. However, humans can take in foods to replace that folate, so the antibiotic is selectively harmful to the bacteria. While all the medicines end in azole, a-z-o-l-e, aripiprazole is a second-generation antipsychotic; its proper stem is -piprazole. Esomeprazole is a proton pump inhibitor used in GERD with a prazole stem. Fluconazole is an azole antifungal and the complete stem is -conazole. Be careful when you see endings that match; make sure you know the actual stem.

QUESTION 14: ANTIBIOTIC SPECTRUMS

We expect that a prescriber who had to order a culture for an antibiotic treatment would likely prescribe a _____ spectrum antimicrobial and then move to a _____ spectrum once the organism is known.

a) Broad, narrow
b) Narrow, broad
c) Short, tall
d) Tall, short

Question 14: Antibiotic Spectrums

We expect that a prescriber who had to order a culture for an antibiotic treatment would likely prescribe a _____ spectrum antimicrobial and then move to a _____ spectrum once the organism is known.

    a) Broad, narrow
    b) Narrow, broad
    c) Short, tall
    d) Tall, short

Answer: A.Broad and narrow. *When an infection is from an unknown organism, we treat it with broad-spectrum antibiotics to cover most possibilities. In the meantime, we order cultures to figure out which organism is causing the infection in order to better treat it. Then, if a narrow-spectrum antibiotic is appropriate we make the switch.*

QUESTION 15: SUPER INFECTIONS

A subclinical infection is below the radar; that is the infection lacks signs or symptoms. However, a superinfection would most likely present as all of the following except:

a) *Clostridium difficile*
b) Oral thrush
c) Otitis media
d) Vaginal *candidiasis*

Question 15: Super Infections

A subclinical infection is below the radar; that is the infection lacks signs or symptoms. However, a superinfection would most likely present as all of the following except:

a) *Clostridium difficile*
b) Oral thrush
c) **Otitis media**
d) Vaginal *candidiasis*

Answer: C. Otitis media is a middle ear infection common in children; the words literally mean ear + inflammation + middle. However, *Clostridium difficile*, oral thrush, and vaginal candidiasis are all examples of potential superinfections that occur after another infection.

QUESTION 16: ANTIBIOTIC RESISTANCE

Sometimes there aren't many choices when treating a
certain pathogen. MRSA is such a concern because it
generally shows resistance to all of the following except:

a) Amoxicillin
b) Cephalexin
c) Ceftriaxone
d) Vancomycin

Question 16: Antibiotic Resistance

Sometimes there aren't many choices when treating a certain pathogen. MRSA is such a concern because it generally shows resistance to all of the following except:

a) Amoxicillin
b) Cephalexin
c) Ceftriaxone
d) **Vancomycin**

Answer: D. Vancomycin. Methicillin-resistant Staphylococcus aureus (MRSA) shows resistance to penicillins like amoxicillin and cephalosporins except those in the fifth generation. Cephalexin is a first-generation cephalosporin and ceftriaxone is a third-generation cephalosporin, so these wouldn't work on MRSA.

QUESTION 17: BETA-LACTAM ANTIBIOTICS

We might hear the term beta-lactam antibiotic as it relates to enzymes and resistance. Which of the following is not a beta-lactam antibiotic?

a) Amoxicillin
b) Cefepime
c) Cephalexin
d) Vancomycin

Question 17: Beta-Lactam Antibiotics

We might hear the term beta-lactam antibiotic as it relates to enzymes and resistance. Which of the following is not a beta-lactam antibiotic?

a) Amoxicillin
b) Cefepime
c) Cephalexin
d) **Vancomycin**

Answer: D. Vancomycin is a glycopeptide that does not contain a beta-lactam ring. Both penicillins like amoxicillin and cephalosporins such as cefepime and cephalexin belong to the class known as beta-lactam antibiotics. This matters because some bacteria excrete beta-lactamase, an enzyme that can destroy the beta-lactam ring making the antibiotic useless.

QUESTION 18: BETA-LACTAMASE INHIBITORS

Sometimes a component of a drug combination has little therapeutic value; rather it provides protection to help the other component work. Which of the following is a protector against beta-lactamase attack?

a) Amoxicillin
b) Azithromycin
c) Cephalexin
d) Clavulanate

Question 18: Beta-Lactamase Inhibitors

Sometimes a component of a drug combination has little therapeutic value; rather it provides protection to help the other component work. Which of the following is a protector against beta-lactamase attack?

a) Amoxicillin
b) Azithromycin
c) Cephalexin
d) Clavulanate

Answer: D. Clavulanate is a beta-lactamase inhibitor that prevents the action of a beta-lactamase, allowing an antibiotic like amoxicillin to work. Beta-lactamase is an enzyme developed by resistant bacteria that inactivates beta-lactam antibiotics. So, if a patient has amoxicillin alone as a pencillin antibiotic, it may not work. But adding clavulanate is much like giving amoxicillin a body guard to protect it from attack. Azithromycin is a macrolide antibiotic and cephalexin is a first-generation cephalosporin.

QUESTION 19: DRUG RESISTANCE

A child presents with an ear infection; however, he has already been on a week-long course of amoxicillin. Which of the following would likely be a reasonable therapeutic option?

a) Amoxicillin for another week
b) Amoxicillin / clavulanate
c) Cephalexin
d) First generation cephalosporin

Question 19: Drug Resistance

A child presents with an ear infection; however, he has already been on a week-long course of amoxicillin. Which of the following would likely be a reasonable therapeutic option?

a) Amoxicillin for another week
b) Amoxicillin / clavulanate
c) Cephalexin
d) First generation cephalosporin

Answer: B. Amoxicillin with clavulanate. This patient has an ear infection that hasn't gone away after a 1-week course of a beta-lactam antibiotic. The patient's infection is likely resistant and producing beta-lactamase. Clavulanate will block beta-lactamase, allowing the amoxicillin to kill the infection. The other options are beta-lactam antibiotics that will not work on a resistant microbe producing beta-lactamase.

QUESTION I10: CEPHALOSPORIN GENERATIONS

When a new drug comes out and it's in a higher generation, we expect it to be better than the last. As we move up the generations with cephalosporins from 1st through 4th we expect to see all of the following except _____.

a) Better Gram- coverage
b) Better Gram+ coverage
c) Better CSF penetration
d) Better Beta-lactamase resistance

Question 110: Cephalosporin Generations

When a new drug comes out and it's in a higher generation, we expect it to be better than the last. As we move up the generations with cephalosporins from 1st through 4th we expect to see all of the following except _____.

a) Better Gram- coverage
b) **Better Gram+ coverage**
c) Better CSF penetration
d) Better Beta-lactamase resistance

Answer: B. Better Gram + coverage. As we move up the cephalosporin generations 1st through 4th, we see better gram-negative coverage, better CSF penetration, and better beta-lactamase resistance. Gram-positive coverage will either remain the same or decrease. [[[Repeat slide do not read]]]

QUESTION I11: MRSA COVERAGE

While cephalosporins have traditionally not had MRSA coverage, this medicine can provide effectiveness:

a) Cephalexin
b) Ceftriaxone
c) Cefepime
d) Ceftaroline

Question 111: MRSA Coverage

While cephalosporins have traditionally not had MRSA coverage, this medicine can provide effectiveness:

a) Cephalexin
b) Ceftriaxone
c) Cefepime
d) Ceftaroline

Answer: D. Only the 5th generation cephalosporin ceftaroline has coverage for MRSA. First generation cephalexin, third-generation ceftriaxone and fourth generation cefepime do not cover MRSA. **[[[Repeat slide do not read]]]**

QUESTION 112: RED MAN SYNDROME

Red man syndrome is something that can be prevented by infusing over 60 minutes. We might expect which of the following to be the culprit if on a patient's chart it does not happen?

a) Azithromycin
b) Clarithromycin
c) Clindamycin
d) Vancomycin

Question 112: Red Man Syndrome

Red man syndrome is something that can be prevented by infusing over 60 minutes. We might expect which of the following to be the culprit if on a patient's chart it does not happen?

a) Azithromycin
b) Clarithromycin
c) Clindamycin
d) Vancomycin

Answer: D. Vancomycin is notorious as the cause of Red Man Syndrome, a serious hypersensitivity reaction that results in rash, redness, and swelling all over the patient's body. None of the other antibiotics listed have this same risk.

QUESTION 113: ANTIBIOTIC CHELATION

Multivalent cations form complexes or chelate with tetracyclines rendering them ineffective. All of the following represent a multivalent cation except: _____.

a) Iron
b) Magnesium
c) Milk
d) Sodium

Question 113: Antibiotic Chelation

Multivalent cations form complexes or chelate with tetracyclines rendering them ineffective. All of the following represent a multivalent cation except: _____.

a) Iron
b) Magnesium
c) Milk
d) **Sodium**

Answer: D. Sodium is a monovalent cation as it only has a +1 charge, and it does not chelate with tetracyclines.
Multivalent cations are ones with a +2 or +3 charge such as iron, aluminum, magnesium, or calcium (which is found in milk).

QUESTION I14: ANTIBIOTIC RESISTANCE

Sometimes there are therapeutic choices that make absolutely no sense. A drug that, by definition, would be ineffective against VRE includes:

a) Ampicillin
b) Doxycycline
c) Linezolid
d) Vancomycin

Question 114: Antibiotic Resistance

Sometimes there are therapeutic choices that make absolutely no sense. A drug that, by definition, would be ineffective against VRE includes:

    a) Ampicillin
    b) Doxycycline
    c) Linezolid
    d) Vancomycin

Answer: D. Vancomycin. VRE stands for vancomycin-resistant enterococci. Definitionally, this microbe is resistant to vancomycin, so vancomycin would be ineffective against it.

QUESTION I15: DURATION OF ACTION

When choosing a therapeutic option, determining how few tablets often helps make the decision easier. Which of the following medications would likely have the fewest doses per day?

a) Amoxicillin
b) Azithromycin
c) Clarithromycin
d) Erythromycin

Question 115: Duration of Action

When choosing a therapeutic option, determining how few tablets often helps make the decision easier. Which of the following medications would likely have the fewest doses per day?

a) Amoxicillin
b) **Azithromycin**
c) Clarithromycin
d) Erythromycin

Answer: B. Azithromycin has the longest duration of action of the macrolides, so it is only dosed once daily. A double dose on the first day, then a daily single dose of four is the most common dosage. Clarithromycin is dosed twice daily, and erythromycin is dosed 4 times daily. Amoxicillin is a beta-lactam antibiotic, and it is dosed 2 to 3 times daily.

QUESTION I16: ANTIFUNGAL MEDICATIONS

Some antifungal medications are only used systemically, and some antifungals are only used on superficial infections. Which of the following antifungal medications can be used for both systemic and superficial infections?

a) Amphotericin B
b) Butenafine
c) Fluconazole
d) Nystatin

Question 116: Antifungal Medications

Some antifungal medications are only used systemically, and some antifungals are only used on superficial infections. Which of the following antifungal medications can be used for both systemic and superficial infections?

a) Amphotericin B
b) Butenafine
c) **Fluconazole**
d) Nystatin

Answer: C. Fluconazole can be used for both systemic and superficial infections. It acts on the inside of fungal membranes and because it is only taken in by fungal cells, it leads to less systemic toxicity. Amphotericin B is used for serious systemic infections. Butenafine and nystatin are used only for superficial infections such as athlete's foot and thrush, respectively.

QUESTION I17: ANTIMYCOBACTERIAL MEDICATIONS

Tuberculosis is a condition that is treated with three to four different medications at the same time to prevent resistance against any one medication. Which of the following medications is not used in the setting of tuberculosis?

a) Rifampin
b) Isoniazid
c) Pyrazinamide
d) Erythromycin

Question 117: Antimycobacterial Medications

Tuberculosis is a condition that is treated with three to four different medications at the same time to prevent resistance against any one medication. Which of the following medications is not used in the setting of tuberculosis?
   a) Rifampin
   b) Isoniazid
   c) Pyrazinamide
   d) Erythromycin

Answer: D. Erythromycin. Tuberculosis medications can be remembered using the acronym RIPE: R, rifampin, I, isoniazid, P, pyrazinamide, and E, ethambutol. You might think of the RIPE positive TB skin test to remember. Erythromycin is not the E in that acronym.

QUESTION 118: ANTIVIRAL TARGETS

Antivirals have a number of processes they can target with their action. Which of the following is not a target for antiviral medications?

a) Viral motility
b) Viral attachment and entry
c) Viral release
d) Nucleic acid synthesis

Question 118: Antiviral Targets

Antivirals have a number of processes they can target with their action. Which of the following is not a target for antiviral medications?

a) **Viral motility**
b) Viral attachment and entry
c) Viral release
d) Nucleic acid synthesis

Answer: A. Viral motility is not targeted by antivirals. Palivizumab targets viral attachment and entry. Acyclovir and valacyclovir target nucleic acid synthesis. Oseltamivir and zanamivir target viral release.

QUESTION I19: ANTIVIRAL MEDICATIONS

Different antiviral medications are used for different conditions. Which of the following medications is used to treat herpes simplex virus (HSV)?

a) Palivizumab
b) Valacyclovir
c) Oseltamivir
d) Ciprofloxacin

Question 119: Antiviral Medications

Different antiviral medications are used for different conditions. Which of the following medications is used to treat herpes simplex virus (HSV)?

a) Palivizumab
b) Valacyclovir
c) Oseltamivir
d) Ciprofloxacin

Answer: B. Valacyclovir is an antiviral medication for HSV and VZV (Varicella-zoster virus). Palivizumab is a monoclonal antibody for respiratory syncytial virus (RSV). Oseltamivir treats influenza, and ciprofloxacin is a fluoroquinolone antibiotic, not an antiviral.

QUESTION 120: HIV ANTIVIRAL MEDICATIONS

HIV antiviral medications target one of ten steps in the HIV replication process. Which of the following steps does the CCR5 antagonist maraviroc (Selzentry) target?

a) Step 1: Attachment
b) Step 2: Fusion
c) Step 5: Integration
d) Step 10: HIV protease processing

Question 120: HIV Antiviral Medications

HIV antiviral medications target one of ten steps in the HIV replication process. Which of the following steps does the CCR5 antagonist maraviroc (Selzentry) target?

a) Step 1: Attachment
b) **Step 2: Fusion**
c) Step 5: Integration
d) Step 10: HIV protease processing

Answer: B. Step 2: Fusion. CCR5 antagonists and fusion inhibitors target step 2: infusion. The integrase strand inhibitor raltegravir targets step 5: integration. The protease inhibitor darunavir targets step 10: HIV protease processing. No HIV antivirals target step 1: attachment.

CHAPTER 5 NEURO

I. OTC Local anesthetics and antivertigo

There are two major classes of local anesthetics named after the molecules in the middle of their structures: esters and amides. Esters, such as **benzocaine (Anbesol),** are generally found in topical agents because when given by injection, they are more allergenic (cause allergic reactions). Amides are less allergenic, therefore, **lidocaine**, an amide, is usually well tolerated when injected. Most students know of **cocaine** and remember these amides are local anesthetics through the "–caine" ending association among the three names: **benzocaine**, **lidocaine**, and cocaine. The over-the-counter (OTC) antiemetic / motion sickness medicine **meclizine (Dramamine)** also has a brand name **Antivert**, for anti-vertigo, which helps memorization.

Local anesthetics – Ester type

Benzocaine (Anbesol)
BEN-zoh-cane (ANN-buh-sawl)

> The "–caine" stem indicates **benzocaine** is a local anesthetic. **Anbesol** numbs an aching tooth.

Local anesthetics – Amide type

Lidocaine (Solarcaine)
LIE-doe-cane (SOH-ler-cane)

Lidocaine is often used topically and is available over-the-counter to treat sunburns, hence the brand name **Solarcaine.** Injectable and patch forms of **lidocaine** are also available by prescription. Paramedics often use **lidocaine** for arrhythmias in emergencies as an injectable, which is part of the L-E-A-N acronym for the emergency medicines: <u>l</u>idocaine, <u>e</u>pinephrine, <u>a</u>tropine, and <u>n</u>aloxone.

ANTIVERTIGO

Meclizine (Dramamine)
MECK-luh-zeen (DRAH-mah-mean)

You can also see "i-z-i-n" from d<u>izzin</u>ess in the generic name **mec<u>lizin</u>e. Antivert** is another brand name of the **<u>antivert</u>**igo drug **meclizine.**

II. SEDATIVE-HYPNOTICS (SLEEPING PILLS)

A patient came into the pharmacy saying his wife wanted **Tylenol PM,** but saw how expensive the brand name product was. I told him that **Tylenol PM** contains **acetaminophen** and **diphenhydramine** and that he could buy both generics separately and it could be cheaper. He thought about it a minute and said, "It might be a little cheaper at first, but when my wife sends me back to get **Tylenol PM,** what she asked for, it might not be cheaper after all." This story highlights the importance of reading OTC labels closely. It's an opportunity for practitioners to help patients understand OTC products.

Sedative-hypnotics like **diphenhydramine** help patients sleep. Most prescription sedative-hypnotics provide hints about their function in their brand names: **Eszopiclone**

(**Lunesta**) contains Luna for "moon," **ramelteon (Rozerem)** refers to REM sleep, and **zolpidem (Ambien)** creates an "ambient" (tranquil) environment.

Although benzodiazepines such as **clonazepam (Klonopin)**, **diazepam (Valium)**, and **lorazepam (Ativan)** work as sedative hypnotics, I discuss benzos later in this chapter as they have other functions as well.

OTC - Non-narcotic analgesic / Sedative-hypnotic

Acetaminophen/Diphenhydramine (Tylenol PM)
uh-seat-uh-MIN-no-fin / dye-fen-HIGH-dra-mean
(TIE-len-all pee em)

> It's common to combine two drugs like **acetaminophen** for aches and **diphenhydramine**, a sedating 1st- generation antihistamine. One of my students came up with take both "phens" when you want to end up sleepin'.

Benzodiazepine-like

Eszopiclone (Lunesta)
es-zo-PEH-clone (Lou-NES-tuh)

> **Eszopiclone's** generic stem "-clone" will put you in the sleeping zone. Some students point to the "z" in **eszopiclone** for getting your z's. The brand name **Lunesta** uses the Latin for moon (Luna) plus part of the word "rest," which makes it memorable.

Zolpidem (Ambien, Ambien CR)
zole-PEH-dem (AM-bee-en)

Use the "-pidem" stem to remember **zolpidem** as a sedative-hypnotic. Some students match the brand name **Ambien** with an ambient, sleepy environment. Controlled Release **zolpidem, Ambien CR**, works for people who have difficulty maintaining sleep (DMS) *and* those who have difficulty falling asleep (DFA). The regular version only works for those with DFA.

MELATONIN RECEPTOR AGONIST

Ramelteon (Rozerem)
ra-MEL-tee-on (row-ZER-em)

The "–melteon" stem in **ramelteon** lets you know it's a melatonin agonist. Another student said the "m-e-l" in **ramelteon** reminded her of mellow. In **Rozerem**, you can see the "z" for z's, the "r-e-m" for REM (rapid eye movement) sleep. Also, "roze" rhymes with doze.

III. ANTIDEPRESSANTS

Antidepressant classes often intimidate students, so let's take them one word at a time. The selective serotonin reuptake inhibitors (SSRIs) class includes drugs such as **citalopram (Celexa), escitalopram (Lexapro), sertraline (Zoloft), paroxetine (Paxil),** and **fluoxetine (Prozac)**. These medications will selectively inhibit reuptake (breakdown) of serotonin within neurons. Increased serotonin levels can improve mood. Note: **escitalopram** has the same "es" prefix (added onto **citalopram**) discussed with the PPIs **esomeprazole** and **omeprazole** where the sinister "S" form is superior.

Similar to the SSRIs are the serotonin-norepinephrine reuptake inhibitors (SNRIs) **duloxetine (Cymbalta)** and **venlafaxine (Effexor)**. Be careful - **duloxetine** is an SNRI, yet has the "–oxetine" stem of some SSRIs **(fluoxetine, paroxetine)**.

SSRIs and SNRIs carry the names of the neurotransmitters they affect. The tricyclic antidepressant (TCA) class name comes from the chemical structure's three rings. **Amitriptyline (Elavil)** is an example**.**

The last group of antidepressants includes the monoamine oxidase inhibitors (MAOIs). A word that ends in "ase" is usually an enzyme, so if an antidepressant blocks the enzyme that breaks a neurotransmitter down, then there is more neurotransmitter (the monoamines, in this case) available to elevate the patient's mood. An example of an MAOI is **isocarboxazid** (**Marplan**).

SELECTIVE SEROTONIN REUPTAKE INHIBITORS (SSRIs)

Citalopram (Celexa)
si-TAL-oh-pram (sell-EX-uh)

> Most students, when seeing two drugs with the same root, **citalopram** and **escitalopram**, quickly put them into long-term memory. One student's trick was to remember that the "p-r-a-m" medications are for de–p–r–ession, but "pram" is not an official stem. I associate the brand name **Celexa** with the word "relax."

Escitalopram (Lexapro)
es-si-TAL-oh-pram (LECKS-uh-pro)

> **Lexapro** takes the last four letters of **Celexa** and adds "pro." You can think of this as the pro-

fessional upgrade, as **Lexapro** came after **Celexa**. It's common for an S isomer to come to market after the original drug has become available as a generic.

Ser<u>traline</u> (Zoloft)
SIR-tra-lean" (ZO-loft)

One should use the "-traline" stem to remember **ser<u>traline</u>** is an SSRI, but most students also memorize the brand name **Zoloft** as "<u>loft</u>ing" a depressed patient's mood.

Flu<u>oxetine</u> (Prozac, Sarafem)
flue-OX-uh-teen (PRO-Zack)

Fluoxetine was the first SSRI to make it to market. The "–oxetine" ending is supposed to be for **fluoxetine**-like entities, but you will see "-oxetine" on the SNRI **dul<u>oxetine</u>** (**Cymbalta**) and ADHD medication **atom<u>oxetine</u>** (**Strattera**), so be careful.

When **fluoxetine** gained a new indication, for premenstrual dysphoric disorder (PMDD), it also gained a new brand name: **Sarafem** – "Sara" like the girl's name and "fem" for feminine. The highest ranked angels are Sera-p-h-i-m, so combatting PMDD is the work of angels.

I don't know if that's what the drug manufacturer was going for. In addition, by taking a new brand name for another indication, it might have prevented the potential confusion of a patient with depression on **Prozac** and a patient with PMDD on **Sarafem**. The combination of "pro" for positive and the strong sounding "zac" ending makes **Prozac** sound like a strong antidepressant.

Paroxetine (Paxil, Paxil CR)
par-OX-eh-teen (PACKS-ill)

> **Paroxetine** is similar to the SSRI **fluoxetine** with the same "–oxetine" stem. **Paxil** takes "p-a-x-"" from **pa**roxetine. The controlled-release CR version of **Paxil** is supposed to have fewer initial side effects and be a little easier to dose.

MISCELLANOUS/ SSRI

Vilazodone (Viibryd)
Vuh-LAYZ-uh-done (VIE-brid)

> **Vilazodone (Viibryd)** is a selective serotonin reuptake inhibitor with partial agonism at the 5-HT_{1A} receptor. After a patient takes Viibryd, they are supposed to be no longer depressed and more vibrant.

SEROTONIN-NOREPINEPHRINE REUPTAKE INHIBITORS (SNRIs)

Duloxetine (Cymbalta)
doo-LOX-eh-teen (SIM-bal-tah)

> **Duloxetine** affects serotonin and norepinephrine and one can think of the "du" as duo (two). I have never seen an unhappy cymbal player in a band and "alta" means tall. Students can use either mnemonic to remember **Cymbalta** elevates mood.

Desvenlafaxine (Pristiq)
des-ven-luh-FAX-een (prih-STEEK)

Desvenlafaxine (Pristiq) is the enantiomer of
venlafaxine (Tranxene).

Venla<u>faxine</u> (Effexor)
ven-luh-FAX-een (Eff-ECKS-or)

This drug is best memorized by its stem "-faxine." If
you look at the "afax" in **venlafaxine** and "Effex" in
Effexor, you can see some commonalities.
Desvenla<u>faxine</u> (Pristiq), in the "Memorizing 350
Drugs" chapter is an SNRI also.

TRICYCLIC ANTIDEPRESSANTS (TCAS)

Ami<u>triptyline</u> (Elavil)
ah-meh-TRIP-tuh-lean (ELLE-uh-vill)

Using the "tri" in **ami<u>triptyline</u>** helps students
remember this is a "T-C-A," or tricyclic
antidepressant. It "trips" up depression. Think of
the brand **Elavil** as <u>elev</u>ating the patient's mood.

Doxe<u>pin</u> (Sinequan)
DAWK-suh-pin (SIN-eh-kwan)

Just note doxepin lacks that normal -triptyline stem
you might be used to with TCAs. The brand looks a
lot like a Latin expression sine qua non, which in
medicine means that if it's not there, that's a good
thing. So, my thought was the brand name came
from thinking once this medicine is in place, the
condition, depression, becomes absent.

Nor<u>triptyline</u> (Pamelor)
nor-TRIP-tuh-lean (Pam-eh-lore)

Using the "tri" in **nor<u>tri</u>ptyline** also helps students remember this is a tricyclic antidepressant. It "trips" up depression. Nortriptyline's effect is stronger on norepinephrine, hence the nor, n-o-r in the name.

TETRACYCLIC ANTIDEPRESSANT (TECA) NORADRENERGIC AND SPECIFIC SEROTONERGIC ANTIDEPRESSANTS (NASSAS)

Mirtazapine (Remeron)
mihr-TAZ-uh-peen (REM-uhr-on)

> **Mirtazapine (Remeron)** is a noradrenergic and specific serotonergic antidepressant (NaSSA).

MONOAMINE OXIDASE INHIBITOR (MAOI)

Isocarboxazid (Marplan)
iso-car-BOX-uh-zid (MAR-plan)

> A student came up with **Marplan** for the atypical sad man who laments, "I so carve boxes" for **isocarboxazid**. In addition, I can take the "m" and "a" from **Marplan** to remember it's an M-A-O-I.

IV. SMOKING CESSATION

There are many nicotine replacement products on the market. I've chosen to focus on two tablets used by prescription that help patients quit smoking: **bupropion (Wellbutrin, Zyban)** and **varenicline (Chantix)**.

Bupropion (Wellbutrin, Zyban)

byou-PRO-pee-on (well-BYOU-trin, ZY-ban)

> **Bupropion** was first marketed as **Wellbutrin**, an atypical antidepressant, one that didn't fit into the SSRIs, SNRIs, TCAs, or MAOIs. Reports must have come in that patients stopped smoking while taking it, so the company repackaged the drug with a new brand name as **Zyban**, to put a "ban" on smoking. There is some risk with this medication, especially in patients with a history of seizures.

Varenicline (Chantix)
Vah-WREN-eh-clean (CHAN-ticks)

> **Varenicline**, another smoking cessation medication, has caused distressing dreams, suicidal thoughts, and other adverse effects. A student, in a southern drawl, remembered varenicline's generic name by saying, "With **varenicline**, 'I'm vary incline ta quit.'" Another came up with "My chant is, 'I don't need my fix' with **Chantix**."

V. BARBITURATES AND BENZODIAZEPINES

Barbiturates are the much less safe version of the benzodiazepines, but I wanted to include **phenobarbital (Luminal)** for completeness. The big concern is respiratory depression.

Benzodiazepines relieve anxiety, insomnia and muscle spasms. Like the tricyclic antidepressants, benzodiazepines get their name from their chemical structure: a benzene ring and a diazepine ring. Because benzodiazepine has many syllables, most people call them benzos. Examples include **alprazolam (Xanax), clonazepam (Klonopin), diazepam**

(**Valium**), and **lorazepam (Ativan)**. Note benzodiazepines have the similar generic suffixes "–azolam" and "–azepam."

BARBITURATES

Pheno<u>barbi</u>tal (Luminal)

> Benzos replaced barbiturates as a sleep aid because barbiturates can cause respiratory depression. A student remembered this by thinking of barbiturates (barbs) as literal barbs on razor wire fences that puncture lungs.

BENZODIAZEPINES

Clon<u>azepam</u> (Klonopin)
kloe-NAZ-uh-pam (KLON-uh-pin)

> **Clonazepam** should be remembered from the "–azepam" stem. The brand name **Klonopin** uses the phonetic spelling of generic **clonazepam's** first four letters "c-l-o-n." Benzos replaced barbiturates as a sleep aid because barbiturates can cause respiratory depression. A student remembered this by thinking of barbiturates (barbs) as literal barbs on razor wire fences that puncture lungs.

Alpr<u>azolam</u> (Xanax)
Al-PRAY-zo-lam (ZAN-ax)

> You should remember benzodiazepines by their two endings, "–azolam" or "–azepam." Be careful as a number of online and highly regarded test prep resources, including those by licensed professionals, refer to benzodiazepine stems as "–pam" or "–lam." That is incorrect. This will lead you to think drugs

that are not benzos are in the class. For example, **verapamil (Calan)** is a calcium channel blocker and **lamotrigine (Lamictal)** is an antiepileptic. I've even seen a well-regarded resource indicate that **citalopram** has a –pam suffix at the end, and that's understandable as some patients drop the "r," pronouncing it "citalo-pam," but this is incorrect. **Alprazolam** has one z; benzodiazepine has two; **Xanax** sounds like a "z" to help you get a snooze and "x's" out anxiety too. You can also look at the word **Xanax** and see the "a-n-x" from anxiety.

Lorazepam (Ativan)
lore-A-zeh-pam (AT-eh-van)

Remember **lorazepam** through the "–azepam" stem or think about the brand name **Ativan** vanquishing anxiety.

Midazolam (Versed)
meh-DAZE-oh-lam (VER-said)

You should remember **midazolam** through the "-azolam" stem, but there are other tips you can use. There are two m's in **midazolam** for the memories you can't form since **midazolam** causes anterograde amnesia. Just as your *ante*brachium is your forearm, and the *ante* is the money poker players put out before the dealer deals, *ante*rograde amnesia is the inability to form memories. Alternatively, you can use the brand name; I can't remember the "verse you just said" for **Versed**.

Temazepam (Restoril)
Tuh-MAY-zuh-pam(RES-tuh-rill)

Temazepam (Restoril) is a benzodiazepine marketed for sleep disorders, i.e. for "<u>rest</u>" or "<u>resto</u>ration."

VI. NON-BENZODIAZEPINES/ NON-BARBITURATE

Bu<u>spiro</u>ne (Buspar)
byou-SPIH-rone (BYOU-spar)

Just as nonfiction literature is classified as "not" fiction, **buspirone (Buspar)** is classified as a non-barbiturate, non–benzodiazepine.

VII. ADHD MEDICATIONS

ADHD (attention-deficit-hyperactivity disorder) stimulants calm a patient who has a hyperactive mind and / or body without a sedative effect. Examples include the drugs **dexmethylphenidate (Focalin)** and **methylphenidate (Concerta)**. These two medications have the same root, **methylphenidate**. In chemistry, compounds direct plane-polarized light to either the left or right. These terms are "d" or "(+)" for dextrorotatory compounds rotating plane-polarized light to the right, or "l" or "(-)" for levorotatory compounds rotating plane-polarized light to the left. **Dexmethylphenidate** rotates plane-polarized light to the right. **Dexmethylphenidate** should be more effective, last longer, and have fewer side effects than methylphenidate.

Atomoxetine (Strattera) is a non-stimulant medication and because there's not a potential for abuse, it doesn't carry a DEA schedule. It's *not* an SSRI like **fluoxetine**, even though it ends in "–oxetine."

STIMULANT – SCHEDULE II

Amphetamine/Dextroamphetamine (Adderall)
Am-FEH-tuh-mean / decks-trow-am-FEH-tuh-mean (ADD-ihr-awl)

> **Adderall** has A-D-D in the name for the attention deficit disorder condition it treats, but when you think about being able to focus, you can now **Adderall**, add 'er all up again, doing math well, in other words.

Dexmethylphenidate (Focalin)
dex-meth-ill-FEN-eh-date (FOE-ca-lin)

> When I was a student, I could remember that **Focalin** and **Concerta** both had **methylphenidate** in their names, but I could never remember which was **dexmethylphenidate** and which was **methylphenidate**. Then I thought of the "F" in "**Focalin**" as following the "d-e" (like in the alphabet) in **dexmethylphenidate** to help me. To remember **Focalin** is for ADHD, you think of **Focalin** helping a patient focus.

Lisdexamfetamine (Vyvanse)
lis-decks-am-FEH-tuh-mean (VIE-vants)

> **Lisdexamfetamine (Vyvanse)** has a British "–fetamine" ending.

Methylphenidate (Ritalin, Concerta)
meth-ill-FEN-eh-date (con-CERT-uh)

> **Methylphenidate** has many brand names, including **Ritalin** and **Concerta.** Most students seem to

already know **methylphenidate,** but remember that
Concerta can help a patient <u>concentrate</u>. To
remember it's an amphetamine, one student said she
thought of staying up all night at a <u>concert</u> with
Concerta. **Concerta** is a long-acting medication that
needs to be taken only once a day.

NON-STIMULANT – NON-SCHEDULED

Atom<u>oxetine</u> (Strattera)
AY-toh-mocks-e-teen (stra-TER-uh)

> Note the "–oxetine" stem here is also not an SSRI
> antidepressant, but a non-stimulant medication for
> ADHD. **Strattera** helps <u>str</u>aighten patients'
> <u>att</u>ention.

IX. BIPOLAR DISORDER

Mood stabilizers such as **lithium** are especially likely to
cause electrolyte imbalances. If you look at the periodic
table, you see that lithium (Li) and sodium (Na) are in the
same group (the alkali metals) and both have a +1 charge as
an ion. Because of this similarity, what happens to sodium
will happen to **lithium,** causing either a toxic or a
subtherapeutic state if too much **lithium** is retained or
excreted, respectively. Other meds, like **risperidone**, can
help control certain symptoms of the disease until the
lithium level is correct.

SIMPLE SALT

Lithium (Lithobid)
LITH-e-um (LITH-oh-bid)

270

Lithium sits in the same group on the periodic table of elements as the Latin *Natrium* (Na), commonly known as the chemical element sodium. The body has trouble telling the difference between lithium and sodium, and too much or too little salt can wreak havoc on **lithium** levels. A way to remember this is the saying, "Where the salt goeth, the **lithium** goeth." The "b-i-d" in the brand name **Lithobid** is the Latin *bis-in-die*, or a twice-daily dosing schedule.

XI. SCHIZOPHRENIA

We break the medication classification for schizophrenia into typical (1st-generation) or atypical (2nd-generation). We further divide the typical antipsychotics **chlorpromazine (Thorazine)** and **Haloperidol (Haldol)** into low potency and high potency, respectively.

While these two antipsychotics have the same therapeutic effects, their side effect profiles are different. Low potency drugs like **chlorpromazine** cause more sedation, but fewer extrapyramidal symptoms. Extrapyramidal symptoms are movement disorders associated with antipsychotics.

High potency drugs like **haloperidol** cause more extrapyramidal symptoms (movement disorders), but less sedation. We prescribe typical antipsychotics for positive symptoms such as delusions, hallucinations and paranoia.

Atypical antipsychotics such as **quetiapine (Seroquel)** and **risperidone (Risperdal)** cause fewer extrapyramidal effects, but have more negative metabolic effects like weight gain, diabetes, and hyperlipidemia. Second-generation drugs work for positive symptoms, such as delusions, as well as negative symptoms, such as poor motivation and emotional and social withdrawal.

FIRST GENERATION ANTIPSYCHOTIC (FGA) LOW POTENCY

Chlorpromazine (Thorazine)
Klor-PRO-mah-zeen (THOR-uh-zeen)

Chlorpromazine was the first antipsychotic. While it carries side effects, it represented a new treatment option for schizophrenic patients. Generational classifications are especially important in antipsychotics because of differences in both side effects and effects on positive versus negative symptoms. Thor is a mythical god, and you can think of **Thorazine** as helping people who have delusions of mythical people.

FIRST GENERATION ANTIPSYCHOTIC (FGA) HIGH POTENCY

Haloperidol (Haldol)
hal-low-PEAR-eh-doll (HAL-doll)

Use the "-peridol" stem to recognize this 1st-generation high potency drug. Many students think of the "halo" in **haloperidol** to remember this is high potency. To make the brand name **Haldol**, they just took the first and last three letters of the generic name **haloperidol**.

SECOND-GENERATION ANTIPSYCHOTICS (SGA) (ATYPICAL ANTIPSYCHOTICS)

Aripiprazole (Abilify)
air-ih-pih-pruh-zole (uh-BIL-uh-fye)

Abilify helps a schizophrenic have more "ability to function in society." The WHO "–piprazole" stem is discouraged because it has the PPI "–prazole" stem in it.

Clozapine (Clozaril)
claw-ZUH-peen (claw-ZUH-rill)

> **Clozapine** requires special testing of white blood cells because of its ability to cause agranulocytosis, a low number of granulocytes, a type of white blood cell. Programs like these are called REMS, or the Clozapine Risk Evaluation and Mitigation Strategy. I love their "no blood, no drug" tagline which can help you remember that blood testing is important.

Olanzapine (Zyprexa)
oh-lan-ZUH-peen (Zie-preck-suh)

> Olanzepine is the safer version of clozapine, but not quite as effective.

Risperidone (Risperdal)
ris-PEAR-eh-done (RIS-per-doll)

> Note the stem "–peridol" from **haloperidol** and "–peridone" from **risperidone** are similar; that can help you remember both of these are antipsychotics. The brand name **Risperdal** and generic name **risperidone** share the opening letters "r-i-s-p-e-r." One student thought of risper and whisper, as in calming the whispering voices.

Quetiapine (Seroquel)
Kweh-TIE-uh-peen (SEAR-uh-kwell)

> In **quetiapine**, you should use the "-tiapine" stem to recognize that this is a 2nd-generation antipsychotic.

If you switch the "i" and "t" in **quetiapine**, you get
the word "quiet," as in quieting the voices.
Seroquel, the brand name, shares the "q-u-e" from
quetiapine and quell means to silence someone.

Ziprasidone (Geodon)
Zih-PRAY-zihd-own (GEE-oh-don)

Use the similarity of **ziprasidone's** -sidone suffix to
risperidone's -peridone suffix to help you
remember these are both second generation
antipsychotics.

XII. ANTIEPILEPTICS

The traditional anti-epileptic drugs **carbamazepine
(Tegretol)**, **divalproex (Depakote)**, and **phenytoin
(Dilantin)** have been around for a long time and we usually
know what to expect with their use.

We may have less experience with the newer anti-epileptics,
such as **gabapentin (Neurontin)** and **pregabalin (Lyrica)**,
but they are often just as effective as the traditional drugs.
Neurologists try medications in a patient until one drug
relieves the seizure symptoms.

TRADITIONAL ANTIEPILEPTICS

Carbamazepine (Tegretol)
car-bah-MAZE-uh-peen (TEG-reh-tawl)

While **carbamazepine's** "-pine," pronounced,
"peen," is the stem, it's not very useful because the –
"-pine" ending just means a chemical has three
rings. Instead, think either of seizures being

"carbed" (curbed) or of being "amazed" that the
seizures are "stopping" using the letters inside **carb-
amaze-pine**. I remember the brand name **Tegretol**
has the "t-r-o-l" in con*trol*, as in to control seizures.

Divalproex (Depakote)
dye-VAL-pro-ex (DEP-uh-coat)

While you can find "v-a-l" in many medication
names, it is helpful to think of the "val" in
di*val*proex and it's similarity with the "v-u-l" in
con*vul*sions. I know it's a stretch. One student
thought of **divalproex** as a <u>pro</u> at <u>ex</u>tracting seizures.

Phenytoin (Dilantin)
FEN-eh-toyn (DYE-lan-tin)

The "–toin" stem helps you remember **pheny<u>toin</u>** is
an antiepileptic. **Dilantin** and shakin' almost rhyme.

NEWER ANTIEPILEPTICS

Gabapentin (Neurontin)
GA-ba-PEN-tin (NER-on-tin)

The "-gab" stem is a little misleading. Neither
<u>gab</u>apentin nor **pre<u>gab</u>alin** directly affect gamma-
amino-butyric-acid (GABA) receptors. However,
having them both have the same stem helps set a
memory device for the newer antiepileptics. The
"neu" in **<u>Neu</u>rontin** is one way to remember that
this is a newer drug.

Lamotrigine (Lamictal)
Luh-moh-trih-jean (luh-MICK-tuhl)

Newer antiepileptics include **lamotrigine (Lamictal),** which has "ictal," meaning seizure.

Levetiracetam (Keppra)
leh-vih-TEER-uh-seat-um (KEP-ruh)

Oxcarbazepine (Trileptal)
oks-car-BAY-zuh-peen (TRY-lept-uhl)

Pregabalin (Lyrica)
pre-GAB-uh-lin (LEER-eh-ca)

> A <u>lyre</u> is a musical instrument, and a <u>lyric</u> is a line in a song. Either way, you can think of a seizure coming back into harmony with **Lyrica.**

Topiramate (Topamax)
toe-PEER-uh-mate (TOE-puh-macks)

XIII. PARKINSON'S, ALZHEIMER'S, MOTION SICKNESS

Most people associate Parkinson's with the celebrity actor Michael J. Fox of *Back to the Future* fame. Using a drug like **levodopa / carbidopa (Sinemet)** for Parkinson's works to restore <u>dopa</u>mine, a neurotransmitter responsible for proper motor function that is seriously depleted by the disease.

Concerning Alzheimer's, I remember vividly calling my grandmother and telling her "I love you," to which she responded, "I hope your wife doesn't find out." There is a cruelty in Alzheimer's, and the patients and their caregivers desperately need your help. A drug like **donepezil** works to restore the neurotransmitter acetylcholine, by reducing its breakdown by acetylcholinesterase.

Benztropine mesylate (Cogentin)
benz-TROW-peen MEH-suh-late (KO-Jen-tin)

> The Parkinson's medication **benztropine mesylate (Cogentin)** hints at <u>cogniti</u>on.

Levo<u>dopa</u> / Carbi<u>dopa</u> (Sinemet)
LEE-vo-doe-pa / CAR-bid-oh-pa" (SIN-uh-met)

> Increased dopamine is critical to dealing with the disease. **Sinemet** combines **levodopa** and **carbidopa** to work synergistically. **Carbidopa** doesn't actually have an antiparkinsonian effect, but it reduces the degradation of **levodopa** so more is available to the patient from a smaller dose.

Selegiline (Eldepryl)
se-LEDGE-eh-lean (EL-duh-pril)

> The "–giline" stem should be your hint that **selegiline** is a Parkinson's medication. You can find the letters of the word senile in the generic name **selegiline**. I used to confuse this as an Alzheimer's medication, but it's not, so I was being a little senile. The brand name **Eldepryl** helps you remember that it relieves symptoms of Parkinson's disease, a condition more prevalent in the "<u>elder</u>ly."

Pramipexole (Mirapex ER)
prah-mih-PECKS-sole (MEER-uh-pecks)

> **Pramipexole (Mirapex)** twists around the generic name

Ropinirole (Requip, Requip XL)

277

row-PIHN-uh-roll (REE-qwip)

> **Ropinirole (Requip)** "<u>equips</u>" a patient to deal with Parkinson's.

ALZHEIMER'S

Donepezil (Aricept)
Doe-NEP-eh-zill (AIR-eh-sept)

> When I think of **donepezil** as an Alzheimer's medication, I think, "I <u>don</u>'t remember <u>zil</u>ch!" The brand name **Aricept** improves per<u>cep</u>tion and Alzheimer's patients' powers of recollection. A student thought of the "air" in **Aricept** as helping a patient who acts somewhat spacey or air-headed.

Memantine (Namenda)
Meh-MAN-teen (Nuh-MEN-duh)

> The generic name **memantine** has "mem" for <u>mem</u>ory in it. The brand name **Namenda** comes from <u>N</u>-<u>M</u>ethyl-<u>D</u>-<u>a</u>spartate **(NMDA)**, the receptor it antagonizes. One of my students always thought of **Namenda** as <u>men</u>ding the brain.

MOTION SICKNESS

Scopolamine (Transderm-Scop)
sco-POL-uh-mean (trans-DERM SCOPE)

> **Transderm-Scop** is a transdermal form of **scopolamine**, for motion sickness. "Trans" means across, "derm" means "skin," so across-the-skin **scopolamine**. It's often used for patients on cruise ships.

278

NERVOUS SYSTEM DRUG QUIZ (LEVEL 1)

Classify these drugs by placing the corresponding drug class letter next to each medication. Try to underline the stems before you start and think about the brand name and function of each drug.

1. Alprazolam (Xanax)
2. Amitriptyline (Elavil)
3. Atomoxetine (Strattera)
4. Citalopram (Celexa)
5. Dexmethylphenidate (Focalin)
6. Divalproex (Depakote)
7. Haloperidol (Haldol)
8. Isocarboxazid (Marplan)
9. Levodopa / Carbidopa (Sinemet)
10. Zolpidem (Ambien)

Nervous System Drug Classes:

A. ADHD drug / non-stimulant
B. ADHD drug / stimulant
C. Antidepressant: MAOI
D. Antidepressant: SNRI
E. Antidepressant: SSRI
F. Antidepressant: TCA
G. Antiepileptic: Newer
H. Antiepileptic: Traditional
I. Antipsychotic: Atypical
J. Antipsychotic: Typical
K. Benzodiazepine
L. Parkinson's
M. Sedative-hypnotic
N. Simple salt

NERVOUS SYSTEM DRUG QUIZ (LEVEL 2)

Classify these drugs by placing the corresponding drug class letter next to each medication. Try to underline the stems before you start and remember the brand name and function of each drug.

1. Venlafaxine
2. Diazepam
3. Phenytoin
4. Quetiapine
5. Isocarboxazid
6. Eszopiclone
7. Fluoxetine
8. Citalopram
9. Selegiline
10. Lithium

Nervous System Drug Classes:

A. ADHD drug/non-stimulant
B. ADHD drug/stimulant
C. Antidepressant: MAOI
D. Antidepressant: SNRI
E. Antidepressant: SSRI
F. Antidepressant: TCA
G. Antiepileptic: Newer
H. Antiepileptic: Traditional
I. Antipsychotic: Atypical
J. Antipsychotic: Typical
K. Benzodiazepine
L. Parkinson's
M. Sedative-hypnotic
N. Simple salt

PRACTICE EXAM PART 5
NEURO/PSYCH

QUESTION NP1: ANTIPSYCHOTIC SIDE EFFECTS

When comparing antipsychotic actions, we are often worried more about side effects because most antipsychotics have a similar efficacy. An antipsychotic notorious for its high risk of extrapyramidal symptoms would include:

a) Chlorpromazine
b) Haloperidol
c) Quetiapine
d) Risperidone

Question NP1: Antipsychotic Side Effects

When comparing antipsychotic actions, we are often worried more about side effects because most antipsychotics have a similar efficacy. An antipsychotic notorious for its high risk of extrapyramidal symptoms would include:

a) Chlorpromazine
b) Haloperidol
c) Quetiapine
d) Risperidone

Answer: B. Haloperidol is notorious for having a high risk of extrapyramidal symptoms. Quetiapine and risperidone are both second-generation antipsychotics (SGA), and they would have a lower risk of extrapyramidal symptoms. Chlorpromazine is a first-generation antipsychotic (FGA), but it is low potency and has a lower risk of extrapyramidal symptoms.

QUESTION NP2: ANTIPSYCHOTIC GENERATIONS

With first generation antipsychotics, potency often correlates to extrapyramidal symptoms (EPS). Which of the following medications would fall under the high potency, first-generation classification?

a) Chlorpromazine
b) Haloperidol
c) Quetiapine
d) Risperidone

Question NP2: Antipsychotic Generations

With first generation antipsychotics, potency often correlates to extrapyramidal symptoms (EPS). Which of the following medications would fall under the high potency, first-generation classification?

a) Chlorpromazine
b) Haloperidol
c) Quetiapine
d) Risperidone

Answer: B. Haloperidol is a high potency FGA. Chlorpromazine is a low potency FGA. Both quetiapine and risperidone are SGAs.

QUESTION NP3: ANTIPSYCHOTIC SIDE EFFECTS

You learn that potency and generation can tell you a lot about an antipsychotic's side-effect profile. You would expect what side effect with chlorpromazine, a low potency 1st generation drug?

a) Extrapyramidal effects
b) Hypercholesterolemia
c) Hyperglycemia
d) Somnolence

Question NP3: Antipsychotic Side Effects

You learn that potency and generation can tell you a lot about an antipsychotic's side-effect profile. You would expect what side effect with chlorpromazine, a low potency 1st generation drug?

a) Extrapyramidal effects
b) Hypercholesterolemia
c) Hyperglycemia
d) Somnolence

Answer: D. Somnolence. Low potency FGAs are known for causing significant drowsiness and moderate extrapyramidal effects. High potency FGAs like haloperidol are more associated with high risk of EPS. Hypercholesterolemia and hyperglycemia are both metabolic side effects that would be associated with use of SGAs like risperidone and quetiapine.

QUESTION NP4: ANTIDEPRESSANT THERAPEUTICS

After a few years of taking paroxetine, a student says, "I've stayed with my part-time job for a year now; I'm sleeping pretty well, and I just feel good about things. Should I keep taking these pills?" You say:

a) I would stop now; I'd say you're cured
b) I'll talk to the prescriber about tapering the dose and we'll evaluate your sleep and mood
c) Let's try a week without them and see if things go badly again
d) No, you need to take these pills for life

Question NP4: Antidepressant Therapeutics

After a few years of taking paroxetine, a student says, "I've stayed with my part-time job for a year now; I'm sleeping pretty well, and I just feel good about things. Should I keep taking these pills?" You say:

a) I would stop now; I'd say you're cured
b) **I'll talk to the prescriber about tapering the dose and we'll evaluate your sleep and mood**
c) Let's try a week without them and see if things go badly again
d) No, you need to take these pills for life

Answer: B. I'll talk to the prescriber about tapering the dose and we'll evaluate your sleep and mood. Antidepressants are a medication that some patients may need to take for life, but not all. It is worth trying to take this patient off this medication. The medication should not be stopped cold as with options A and C; it needs to be properly tapered.

QUESTION NP5: ANTIDEPRESSANT STEMS

A student states in class, "A notecard here says the –oxetine ending always means it's an SSRI antidepressant, but there's another "-oxetine" drug that works as an antidepressant on serotonin and norepinephrine." You answer that _____ is for depression and affects both neurotransmitters.

a) Atomoxetine
b) Duloxetine
c) Fluoxetine
d) Paroxetine

Question NP5: Antidepressant Stems

A student states in class, "A notecard here says the –oxetine ending always means it's an SSRI antidepressant, but there's another "-oxetine" drug that works as an antidepressant on serotonin and norepinephrine." You answer that _____ is for depression and affects both neurotransmitters.

a) Atomoxetine
b) Duloxetine
c) Fluoxetine
d) Paroxetine

Answer: B Duloxetine. -oxetine is a stem that can mean different classes of medications; it does not always mean that it is an SSRI. Fluoxetine and paroxetine are both SSRIs, which means they work only on serotonin. Atomoxetine is a non-stimulant ADHD medication that is not used for depression. Duloxetine is an SNRI, which means that it works on both serotonin and norepinephrine.

QUESTION NP6: ANTIDEPRESSANT MECHANISMS OF ACTION

"How do I know which neurotransmitter an antidepressant affects?" a student asks. "I see serotonin a lot." You answer, "With paroxetine, you definitely affect serotonin. With fluoxetine, the drug affects _____":

a) GABA and norepinephrine
b) Norepinephrine only
c) Serotonin and norepinephrine
d) Serotonin only

Question NP6: Antidepressant Mechanisms of Action

"How do I know which neurotransmitter an antidepressant affects?" a student asks. "I see serotonin a lot." You answer, "With paroxetine, you definitely affect serotonin. With fluoxetine, the drug affects_____":

a) GABA and norepinephrine
b) Norepinephrine only
c) Serotonin and norepinephrine
d) Serotonin only

Answer: D. Fluoxetine is also an SSRI, so it selectively affects serotonin just like paroxetine. SNRIs such as duloxetine and venlafaxine affect both serotonin and norepinephrine. The top two options do not apply to any drugs we have learned.

QUESTION NP7: ANTIDEPRESSANT CLASSES

We name antidepressant drug classes after neurotransmitters, chemical shapes, or enzymatic effect. Which antidepressant below has a drug class that comes from neurotransmitters?

a) Amitriptyline
b) Isocarboxazid
c) Nortriptyline
d) Paroxetine

Question NP7: Antidepressant Classes

We name antidepressant drug classes after neurotransmitters, chemical shapes, or enzymatic effect. Which antidepressant below has a drug class that comes from neurotransmitters?

  a) Amitriptyline
  b) Isocarboxazid
  c) Nortriptyline
  d) Paroxetine

Answer: D. Paroxetine is a selective serotonin reuptake inhibitor (SSRI). This is named for the action it has on the neurotransmitter serotonin. Amitriptyline and nortriptyline are both tricyclic antidepressants (TCAs). The tricyclic portion of the name refers to the chemical shape of the molecules. Isocarboxazid is a monoamine oxidase inhibitor (MAOI), which is named for the enzyme it inhibits.

QUESTION NP8: ANTIDEPRESSANT NAMING

Sometimes the neurotransmitters that a drug affects hide behind an enzymatic effect that catalyzes the reaction. Which of the following antidepressant classes comes from the name of an enzymatic inhibition effect?

a) Amitriptyline
b) Escitalopram
c) Isocarboxazid
d) Sertraline

Question NP8: Antidepressant Naming

Sometimes the neurotransmitters that a drug affects hide behind an enzymatic effect that catalyzes the reaction. Which of the following antidepressant classes comes from the name of an enzymatic inhibition effect?

a) Amitriptyline
b) Escitalopram
c) **Isocarboxazid**
d) Sertraline

Answer: C. Isocarboxazid is a monoamine oxidase inhibitor. It is named for the enzyme monoamine oxidase, which it inhibits. Escitalopram and sertraline are both SSRIs, named for the neurotransmitter they affect. Amitriptyline is a TCA, named for its chemical structure.

QUESTION NP9: ANTIDEPRESSANT ADMINISTRATION

Some foods are high in tyramine, an amino acid that can affect blood-pressure control. Aged cheddar, processed meats, and home brewed beer are some foods that contain large quantities. Therefore, giving _____ as an antidepressant would concern you if a patient had these foods in his or her diet.

a) Escitalopram
b) Isocarboxazid
c) Lorazepam
d) Sertraline

Question NP9: Antidepressant Administration

Some foods are high in tyramine, an amino acid that can affect blood-pressure control. Aged cheddar, processed meats, and home brewed beer are some foods that contain large quantities. Therefore, giving _____ as an antidepressant would concern you if a patient had these foods in his or her diet.

a) Escitalopram
b) Isocarboxazid
c) Lorazepam
d) Sertraline

Answer: B. Isocarboxazid is an MAOI, which is a class that has a serious interaction with tyramine. This interaction can lead to elevated blood pressure in the patient. Escitalopram and sertraline are SSRIs, and lorazepam is a benzodiazepine. None of these drug classes interact with tyramine. **[[[Do not read duplicate slide]]]**

QUESTION NP10: BIPOLAR MEDICATION ADMINISTRATION

You dust off your Periodic Table of Elements because you find that lithium is impacted by cations with a plus-one charge. When a patient on lithium says, "I binge on salty chips every other day," you are especially concerned about this element:

a) Aluminum
b) Calcium
c) Magnesium
d) Sodium

Question NP10: Bipolar Medication Administration

You dust off your Periodic Table of Elements because you find that lithium is impacted by cations with a plus-one charge. When a patient on lithium says, "I binge on salty chips every other day," you are especially concerned about this element:

a) Aluminum
b) Calcium
c) Magnesium
d) Sodium

Answer: D. Sodium is an element with a plus-one charge that would interact with lithium. Aluminum, calcium, and magnesium are elements with a greater than plus-one charge. They would not interact with lithium, though they would interact with tetracycline and fluoroquinolone antibiotics.

QUESTION NP11: SEDATIVE-HYPNOTIC ADMINISTRATION

A schoolteacher says, "I have three kids who just won't go to bed until late. I crash right after they do, but find myself waking up in the middle of the night." He feels sluggish during the day because of this insomnia. Which drug would likely help him sleep through the night?

a) Duloxetine
b) Sertraline
c) Zolpidem
d) Zolpidem CR

Question NP11: Sedative-Hypnotic Administration

A schoolteacher says, "I have three kids who just won't go to bed until late. I crash right after they do, but find myself waking up in the middle of the night." He feels sluggish during the day because of this insomnia. Which drug would likely help him sleep through the night?

    a) Duloxetine
    b) Sertraline
    c) Zolpidem
    d) Zolpidem CR

Answer: D. Zolpidem CR. Duloxetine and sertraline are both antidepressants that actually give energy, so they would not help with sleep issues. Zolpidem is a hypnotic that would help with sleep issues, and it should be given to this patient in its controlled release (CR) form to last through the night.

QUESTION NP12: SHORT-TERM ANXIETY

Long-term anxiety treatment often differs from the more immediate short-term treatment. A medicine that helps with a more immediate anxiety attack might be:

a) Alprazolam
b) Citalopram
c) Escitalopram
d) Sertraline

Question NP12: Short-term Anxiety

Long-term anxiety treatment often differs from the more immediate short-term treatment. A medicine that helps with a more immediate anxiety attack might be:

a) **Alprazolam**
b) Citalopram
c) Escitalopram
d) Sertraline

Answer: A. Alprazolam is a benzodiazepine that acts as an anxiolytic (anti-anxiety) within 60-120 minutes, so it is more useful in this case. Citalopram, escitalopram, and sertraline are all SSRIs that would be useful for a patient with anxiety. However, they take up to 4-6 weeks for full effect, so they are not helpful for a more immediate anxiety attack.

QUESTION NP13: ANTI-ANXIETY AGENTS

A patient with panic disorder fails on fluoxetine and the prescriber wants to try a different mechanism of action. Which drug fits that criteria?

a) Duloxetine
b) Escitalopram
c) Paroxetine
d) Sertraline

Question NP13: Anti-Anxiety Agents

A patient with panic disorder fails on fluoxetine and the prescriber wants to try a different mechanism of action. Which drug fits that criteria?

a) **Duloxetine**
b) Escitalopram
c) Paroxetine
d) Sertraline

Answer A. Duloxetine is an SNRI, which means it affects both serotonin and norepinephrine. Escitalopram, paroxetine, sertraline, and fluoxetine are all SSRIs, which means they all selectively affect serotonin. **[[[Do not read repeat slide]]]**

QUESTION NP14: ADHD AGENTS

A parent says, "The doc told me we might see ghost pills, but my kiddo was just bouncing off the wall and I didn't have time to ask if I caught that right. What does she mean by ghost pills?" You believe she is referring to this stimulant medication's long-acting casing.

a) Alprazolam
b) Atomoxetine
c) Fluoxetine
d) Methylphenidate

Question NP14: ADHD Agents

A parent says, "The doc told me we might see ghost pills, but my kiddo was just bouncing off the wall and I didn't have time to ask if I caught that right. What does she mean by ghost pills?" You believe she is referring to this stimulant medication's long-acting casing.

a) Alprazolam
b) Atomoxetine
c) Fluoxetine
d) Methylphenidate

Answer: D. Methylphenidate is a long-acting stimulant medication used for ADHD. Its long-acting casing will often not be digested properly, causing "ghost pills" to appear in the stool. The medication was still absorbed; it just left the casing behind. Atomoxetine is a nonstimulant ADHD medication. Alprazolam is a benzodiazepine, and fluoxetine is an SSRI. Neither are used to treat ADHD directly.

QUESTION NP15: ADHD PATHOLOGY

Many neurological disorders are associated with deficiencies in specific parts of the brain. ADHD patients tend to have less activity in which part of the brain? It is associated with planning, problem-solving, short-term memory, and behavior.

a) Substantia nigra
b) Hippocampus
c) Prefrontal cortex
d) Motor cortex

Question NP15: ADHD Pathology

Many neurological disorders are associated with deficiencies in specific parts of the brain. ADHD patients tend to have less activity in which part of the brain? It is associated with planning, problem-solving, short-term memory, and behavior.

a) Substantia nigra
b) Hippocampus
c) **Prefrontal cortex**
d) Motor cortex

Answer: C. The prefrontal cortex is the area of the brain affected in ADHD. The substantia nigra is affected in Parkinson's disease, and the hippocampus is affected in Alzheimer's disease. The substantia nigra is a part of the motor cortex, the "gas and break pedal."

QUESTION NP16: PARKINSON'S AGENTS

Sometimes, portions of drugs are not directly active in treating the disease state. Instead, these drugs help to make other portions of the drug work better. Which of the following drugs is used to protect another drug in the treatment of Parkinson's?

a) Levodopa
b) Carbidopa
c) Selegiline
d) Donepezil

Question NP16: Parkinson's Agents

Sometimes, portions of drugs are not directly active in treating the disease state. Instead, these drugs help to make other portions of the drug work better. Which of the following drugs is used to protect another drug in the treatment of Parkinson's?

a) Levodopa
b) Carbidopa
c) Selegiline
d) Donepezil

Answer: B. Carbidopa is a dopa decarboxylase inhibitor. It protects levodopa from being converted to dopamine outside of the brain. Levodopa is the dopamine precursor, and it becomes an active drug after conversion in the brain. Selegiline prevents the breakdown of dopamine in the brain. It is often used alongside carbidopa/levodopa, but it does not provide a protective effect. It acts directly on the Parkinson's itself. Donepezil is a medication used in Alzheimer's, and it is not relevant to this question.

QUESTION NP17: ALZHEIMER'S AGENTS

NDMA receptor antagonists such as memantine act to regulate the levels of a certain ion in neurons. Regulation of this ion is associated with increased learning and memory ability, as well as increased neuron lifespan. Which ion does memantine help to regulate?

a) Sodium
b) Potassium
c) Calcium
d) Magnesium

Question NP17: Alzheimer's Agents

NDMA receptor antagonists such as memantine act to regulate the levels of a certain ion in neurons. Regulation of this ion is associated with increased learning and memory ability, as well as increased neuron lifespan. Which ion does memantine help to regulate?

a) Sodium
b) Potassium
c) Calcium
d) Magnesium

Answer: C. Calcium. When calcium levels in neurons are too high, it is associated with decreased learning/memory and neuronal degradation. Memantine binds to NDMA receptors on neurons, regulating the calcium levels inside.

QUESTION NP18: ANTIEPILEPTIC AGENTS

Sometimes we see antiepileptics like divalproex prescribed for a bipolar indication, but there are reasons to prescribe others. Which of the following is most likely an antiepileptic medication on the chart?

a) Carbamazepine
b) Chlorpromazine
c) Citalopram
d) Cyclobenzaprine

Question NP18: Antiepileptic Agents

Sometimes we see antiepileptics like divalproex prescribed for a bipolar indication, but there are reasons to prescribe others. Which of the following is most likely an antiepileptic medication on the chart?

a) **Carbamazepine**
b) Chlorpromazine
c) Citalopram
d) Cyclobenzaprine

Answer: A. Carbamazepine is an antiepileptic agent that acts by inhibiting sodium channels on hyperactive neurons. Chlorpromazine is a low-potency FGA; citalopram is an SSRI, and cyclobenzaprine is a muscle relaxer.

QUESTION NP19: ALCOHOL PREVENTATIVE MEDICATIONS

Alcoholics are often prescribed medications that will help to prevent relapses. Which of the following medications helps with this by binding to the same sites as alcohol in the CNS, thus preventing the uncomfortable feelings associated with abstinence?
   a) Acamprosate
   b) Naltrexone
   c) Amitriptyline
   d) Disulfiram

Question NP19: Alcohol Preventative Medications

Alcoholics are often prescribed medications that will help to prevent relapses. Which of the following medications helps with this by binding to the same sites as alcohol in the CNS, thus preventing the uncomfortable feelings associated with abstinence?

 a) **Acamprosate**
 b) Naltrexone
 c) Amitriptyline
 d) Disulfiram

Answer: A. Acamprosate acts by binding to the same site as alcohol in the CNS, preventing feelings of discomfort. Naltrexone is also used for alcoholism, and it acts by blocking μ-opioid receptors in the CNS, preventing the euphoria associated with drinking. Disulfiram is also used for alcoholism, and it acts by preventing complete alcohol breakdown, resulting in severe nausea/vomiting should the patient drink. Amitriptyline is a TCA that is not usually used in this setting.

QUESTION NP20: SMOKING CESSATION AIDS

A patient has come into your clinic asking about smoking cessation aids. He also has been diagnosed with depression and was wondering which medications might be able to help with both. You know that while varenicline only helps with smoking cessation, bupropion helps:

a) With depression only
b) With smoking cessation only
c) With both depression and smoking cessation
d) With neither condition

Question NP20: Smoking Cessation Aids

A patient has come into your clinic asking about smoking cessation aids. He also has been diagnosed with depression and was wondering which medications might be able to help with both. You know that while varenicline only helps with smoking cessation, bupropion helps:

a) With depression only
b) With smoking cessation only
c) **With both depression and smoking cessation**
d) With neither condition

Answer: C. Bupropion is an atypical antidepressant that is also used in smoking cessation. Varenicline is a partial nicotinic-receptor agonist that will only help with smoking cessation.

CHAPTER 6 CARDIO

I. OTC Antihyperlipidemics and ANTIPLATELET

Few over-the-counter (OTC) medications help a patient with cardiologic issues. Both **Omega-3-acid ethyl esters (Lovaza)** and **Niacin (Niaspan ER)** come as brand name and OTC products, and are used to reduce cholesterol's impact on the patient. Plain **aspirin** (**Ecotrin**) in a low-dose of 81 milligrams helps prevent platelets from clotting, reducing a patient's chance of a heart attack.

OTC Antihyperlipidemics

Omega-3-acid ethyl esters (Lovaza)
Oh-MEG-uh THREE AS-sid ETH-ill EST-ers (Loh-VAH-zah)

> **Omega-3-fatty acids** are available over-the-counter, but there is also a prescription version that undergoes rigorous FDA testing. **Lovaza** is a prescription brand name, but you can find **omega-3-fatty acids** over-the-counter commonly labeled as "Fish Oil."

Niacin (Niaspan ER)
NYE-uh-sin (NYE-uh-span ee-ar)

> A vitamin like **niacin** can reduce cholesterol levels in the body, however it may cause facial flushing that an **aspirin** thirty minutes before treatment prevents.

OTC Antiplatelet

Aspirin (Ecotrin)
AS-per-in (ECK-oh-trin)

> The 81mg daily **aspirin** dosage is not for analgesia or fever reduction. Rather, it keeps platelets from sticking, helping prevent strokes and heart attacks.

II. Diuretics

The order of important structures in the nephron goes from *glomerulus* to *proximal convoluted tubule* (something in close proximity is near) to *Loop of Henle* to *distal convoluted tubule* (something that's distant or distal is far) to the *collecting duct*. The order of diuretics would then be:

1. Osmotic diuretics like **mannitol (Osmitrol)** work at the proximal convoluted tubule (PCT).

2. Loop diuretics like **furosemide (Lasix)** affect the Loop of Henle.

3. Thiazide diuretics like **hydrochlorothiazide (Microzide)** work at the distal convoluted tubule (DCT).

4. Potassium sparing diuretics like **triamterene (Dyrenium)** and **spironolactone (Aldactone)** work at the collecting duct.

Picture a water slide. A lot of water flows at the top (the glomerulus). A trickle flows at the bottom (the collecting duct). Similarly, diuretics produce less diuresis as they continue down the waterslide. The order from most to least diuresis is osmotic > loop > thiazide > potassium sparing.

323

Osmotic

Mannitol (Osmitrol)
MAN-eh-tall (OZ-meh-trawl)

> **Mannitol**, an osmotic diuretic reduces intracranial pressure in an emergency. The brand name **Osmitrol** combines the class of medication "osmotic," and adds that it helps control brain swelling. The actor Bruce Lee died from this event.

Loop

Furosemide (Lasix)
Fyoor-OH-seh-mide (LAY-six)

> Chemists named this class of diuretics after the part of the nephron the drug works in, the Loop of Henle. While the "–semide" stem indicates a "furosemide-type" diuretic, that's like defining a word with the word itself. One student said, "I have to pee furiously" as her mnemonic since loop diuretics produce significant diuresis. The brand name **Lasix** indicates it lasts six hours.

Thiazide

Hydrochlorothiazide (Microzide)
High-droe-klor-oh-THIGH-uh-zide (MY-crow-zide)

> Thiazide diuretics get their class name from the stem of generic drugs like **hydrochlorothiazide**. The abbreviation HCTZ comes from "h" for hydro, "c" for chloro, "t" for thia, and "z" for zide. Thiazides don't produce as much diuresis as loop diuretics, but are excellent for initial treatment of

hypertension. While the "hydro" in **hydrochlorothiazide** stands for the <u>hydro</u>gen atom, you can think of "hydro" as "water" for diuretic. The brand **Microzide** has thia<u>zide</u>'s last four letters.

POTASSIUM SPARING AND THIAZIDE

Triamterene / Hydrochloro<u>thiaz</u>ide (Dyazide)
try-AM-terr-een / High-droe-klor-oh-THIGH-uh-zide (DIE-uh-zyde)

> The combination of a potassium sparing diuretic (**triamterene**) and thiazide (**hydrochlorothiazide**) keeps potassium levels in balance while producing modest diuresis. The brand name **Dyazide** is triamterene's old brand name **Dyrenium** plus the last five letters of **hydrochloro<u>thiaz</u>ide**.

POTASSIUM SPARING

Spironolactone (Aldactone)
spear-oh-no-LACK-tone (Al-DAK-tone)

> **Spironolactone** is another potassium sparing diuretic, but this drug can cause gynecomastia. Gynecomastia is an enlargement of male breasts. To remember **spironolactone** works in the collecting duct, I look at the "lactone," and think "last one." I know a lactone is a kind of chemical structure, but its place of action sticks in my head with this mnemonic.
>
> To come up with the brand name, the manufacturer simply replaced the "spironol" of **spirono<u>lactone</u>** with "ald" to make **<u>Ald</u>actone**. The "ald" is especially important because **spironolactone** blocks

aldosterone, an important steroid hormone that helps the body retain sodium and water when blood pressure drops.

ELECTROLYTE REPLENISHMENT

Potassium chloride (K-Dur)
poe-TASS-ee-um klor-eyed (Kay-Dur)

> **Potassium chloride** is a supplement often administered when a potassium sparing diuretic is contraindicated or when a loop diuretic lowers a patient's potassium levels. The "K" in **K-Dur** is the chemical symbol for potassium. The "Dur" is for long duration.

III. UNDERSTANDING THE ALPHAS AND BETAS

Confusion about alpha-adrenergic antagonists like **doxazosin (Cardura)** and beta-adrenergic antagonists like **propranolol (Inderal)** comes from seeing the receptor names, alpha and beta, instead of drug classifications; e.g., both **doxazosin** and **propranolol** are blood pressure lowering pills.

Alpha and beta are the first two letters of the Greek alphabet and name the receptors where these medications work. An adrenergic *agonist* works *like* adrenaline while an adrenergic *antagonist* works in the *opposite* way.

The prefix "adren" refers to the adrenal glands. The adrenal glands are *above* (ad) the *kidney* (renal) and secrete adrenaline. The suffix "ergic" refers to the Greek for "works like." Therefore, these drugs work like **adrenaline**. Note: **Adrenaline** and **epinephrine** are the same. **Epinephrine** uses the Greek translation of *above* (epi) and *kidney* (neph) to make **epinephrine** instead of the Latin form, **adrenaline**.

Instead of calling a drug a blood pressure pill (antihypertensive), its therapeutic class, prescribers classify a drug by the receptor it affects. By calling **propranolol (Inderal)** a beta-blocker, it's easier not to pigeonhole a drug into one use. Beta-blockers, for example, can treat angina pectoris, congestive heart failure, stage fright, and migraine, in addition to hypertension. **Doxazosin**, the alpha-blocker, also has multiple uses, including hypertension and benign prostatic hyperplasia (BPH). This is why classifying by the receptor name alpha or beta makes more sense.

Furthermore, there are receptor sub-types. Beta-1 receptors are concentrated in the heart (and we have one heart), and beta-2 receptors are concentrated in the lungs (and we have two lungs). You can find them in other places in the body, but for our introductory purposes, it's useful to think in this way.

If a beta-blocker is *non-selective*, like **propranolol (Inderal)**, it can affect both beta-1 receptors in the heart to lower heart rate (good), block beta-2 receptors in the lungs and cause bronchoconstriction (bad). An asthmatic patient might have an adverse reaction to a drug that bronchoconstricts as a side effect.

We prefer **metoprolol (Lopressor)** to control blood pressure because it's selective for just the heart; it's classified as *beta-1 selective*. However, the body will try to compensate for this reduction in blood pressure by vasoconstricting arterioles.

Carvedilol (Coreg), a 3rd-generation beta-blocker, shows that it might be the best choice because it has vasodilating effects to counteract the vasoconstriction as well as cardiac effects.

ALPHA-1 ANTAGONIST

Doxazosin (Cardura)
Docks-AZ-oh-sin (car-DUR-uh)

The blockade of alpha-1 receptors by **doxazosin** causes vasodilation and subsequent reduction in blood pressure. Memorize the stem "–azosin" as an alpha-blocker. You can also link the brand name, as **Cardura** provides durable cardiac relief of hypertension.

Terazosin (Hytrin)
ter-AZ-oh-sin (HIGH-trin)

The cardio drugs are mostly combinations of old drugs. The alpha-1 antagonist **terazosin (Hytrin)** has an "–azosin" ending and **Hytrin** takes six letters from "hypertension."

ALPHA-2 AGONIST

Clonidine (Catapres)
KLAH-neh-deen (CAT-uh-press)

Clonidine works in the brain by affecting alpha-2 receptors to reduce peripheral vascular resistance. You can look at the brand name **Catapres** and think of catabolize (break down) pressure (blood pressure).

Prescribers use **clonidine** in ADHD as single therapy or with stimulants like **methylphenidate (Concerta)**. I had the weirdest experience at the gym. A parent had a loud and lengthy discussion with a psychiatrist about her child's **clonidine** and

Concerta while lifting weights. I never forgot the **clonidine / Concerta** tandem after that.

BETA BLOCKERS – 1ST-GENERATION – NON-BETA-SELECTIVE

Propranolol (Inderal)
Pro-PRAN-uh-lawl (IN-dur-all)

> **Propranolol's** last four letters have the "–olol" beta-blocker stem. The "o-l-o-l" looks like two letter "b's" backwards. Alternatively, if you "oh, laugh out loud," your heart rate goes down from stress relief. If you think of the last "al" in the brand name **Inderal** as it blocks "all" beta-receptors, you can remember this is a non-selective blocker.

BETA BLOCKERS – 2ND-GENERATION – BETA-SELECTIVE

Atenolol (Tenormin)
uh-TEN-oh-lol (Teh-NOR-min)

> While the "–olol" in **atenolol** identifies this medication as a beta-blocker, a student does have to memorize that **atenolol** is 2nd generation. You can do that by memorizing its position after a non-selective first generation **propranolol** in this book or by seeing the "ten" in **atenolol** and knowing it's divisible by two. The "Ten" in the brand name **Tenormin** also matches to the "ten" in **aten**olol.

Atenolol / Chlorthalidone (Tenoretic)
uh-TEN-oh-lol / klor-tha-lih-done (ten-OR-et-ik)

Atenolol with **chlorthalidone** is **Tenoretic**.
Tenoretic takes the "T-e-n-o-r" from **Tenormin** and
adds "r-e-t-i-c" from "diu<u>retic</u>."

Bisopro<u>lol</u> / Hydrochloro<u>thiazide</u> (Ziac)
bih-SEW-pruh-lawl / high-droe-klor-oh-THIGH-uh-zide (ZIE-ak)

> **Bisoprolol (Zebeta)** and **hydrochlorothiazide
> (Microzide)** combine to form **Ziac**.

Metopro<u>lol</u> tartrate (Lopressor)
meh-TOE-pruh-lawl TAR-trait (low-PRESS-or)

> Practitioners rarely highlight the distinction in salts
> like tartrate and succinate, but it's important to
> recognize, as **metoprolol tartrate** and **metoprolol
> succinate** work for different lengths of time.
>
> It would have been nice if the succinate was short
> acting and the tartrate, long acting; then alphabetical
> order would have worked for "s" for short acting.
> That it goes contrary to this logic is how I remember
> which is which. You can use the brand name
> **Lopressor** to remind you that **Lopressor** <u>lo</u>wers
> blood <u>press</u>ure.

Metopro<u>lol</u> succinate (Toprol XL)
meh-TOE-pruh-lawl SUCKS-sin-ate" (TOE-prall ex-ell)

> **Metoprolol succinate** is a long-acting form of
> **metoprolol**. The XL, often used to identify clothing
> as extra-large, indicates an extra-long acting effect in
> medications like **Toprol XL**.

BETA BLOCKERS – 3RD-GENERATION – NON-BETA-SELECTIVE, VASODILATING

Carve<u>dil</u>ol (Coreg)
car-veh-DILL-awl (CO-reg)

> I'm not sure if it was intentional to create a kind of hybrid stem with the "dil" replacing the first "o" in "olol," but you can remember **carvedilol** works by both vasodilation and beta-blockade in this way. The only official stem, however, is the "-dil-." I remember the brand name **Coreg** because it <u>reg</u>ulates <u>cor</u>onary function.

Lab<u>etal</u>ol (Normodyne)
luh-BAY-tuh-lawl (nor-MOH-dyne)

> **Labetalol (Normodyne)** has "<u>beta</u>" in the generic name. Instead of "–olol" for beta-blocker, the stem is –alol for alpha / beta-blocker.

Nebiv<u>olol</u> (Bystolic)
neh-BIH-vuh-lawl (bih-STALL-ick)

> **Nebivolol's** brand name **(Bystolic)** takes letters from sy<u>stolic</u> (the top blood pressure number) and dia<u>stolic</u> (the bottom number).

IV. THE RENIN-ANGIOTENSIN-ALDOSTERONE-SYSTEM DRUGS

The RAAS, or <u>r</u>enin-<u>a</u>ngiotensin-<u>a</u>ldosterone <u>s</u>ystem, controls blood pressure. By defining a few words in this system, we can better understand how the drugs work. The word **renin** comes from **renal** for kidneys, and this enzyme converts angiotensinogen to angiotensin I. Angiotensin converting enzyme (ACE) converts **angiotensin I to angiotensin II**. Angiotensin II is a potent vasoconstrictor and increases blood pressure when that is what our body needs. **Aldosterone** causes the retention of sodium and water, which can further increase blood pressure.

Angiotensin converting enzyme inhibitors (ACE inhibitors) such as **enalapril (Vasotec)** and **lisinopril (Zestril)** stop the body from creating this potent vasoconstrictor, thereby reducing hypertension.

ARBs, or angiotensin II receptor blockers, such as **losartan (Cozaar), olmesartan (Benicar)**, and **valsartan (Diovan)**, block or inhibit the connection between angiotensin II and the receptor that would cause vasoconstriction. This class of drugs is often used as an alternative to an ACE inhibitor when a patient experiences cough as a side effect from an ACE inhibitor.

Here is a mnemonic a student of mine who loved literature made up. It might help you remember the difference: D'artagnan the musketeer has to be "sartan" with the bARB of his blade, otherwise, he'll not be an ACE in April, I'm afraid.

ANGIOTENSIN CONVERTING ENZYME INHIBITORS (ACEIS)

Benazepril / HCTZ (Lotensin HCT)
beh-NAY-zuh-pril (LOW-ten-sin)

> **Benazepril (Lotensin)** becomes **Lotensin HCT** when the manufacturer adds **hydrochlorothiazide, HCTZ**.

Enalapril (Vasotec)
eh-NAL-uh-pril (VA-zo-teck)

Sometimes students simply refer to the ACEIs like **enalapril** as "prils" based on the stem "-pril." While **enalapril** is taken orally, **enalaprilat** is an injectable form and active metabolite of **enalapril**. The brand **Vasotec** alludes to <u>vas</u>odilation on the <u>vas</u>culature.

Fosinopril (Monopril)
foe-SIN-uh-pril (MAW-no-pril)

Fosinopril (Monopril) and Quina<u>pril</u> (Accu<u>pril</u>) are unusual in that the ACE inhibitor stem in both their brand and generic names. Monopril is a mono, or once daily dosing.

Quina<u>pril</u> (Accupril)
KWIN-uh-pril (ah-KYOU-pril)

Lisino<u>pril</u> (Zestril)
lie-SIN-oh-pril (ZES-tril)

Lisinopril, like **enalapril,** works to block the vasoconstricting effects of angiotensin II. A student came up with "**Lisinopril** thrills an overworked heart, blocking angiotensin II from getting a start."

Lisino<u>pril</u> / Hydrochloro<u>thiazide</u> (Zestoretic)
lie-SIN-oh-pril / High-droe-klor-oh-THIGH-uh-zide (ZES-tuh-reh-tik)

When a manufacturer adds **hydrochlorothiazide (Microzide)** to **Lisinopril (Zestril),** it becomes **Zestoretic** by adding the last letters of "diu<u>retic</u>" to the name.

Rami<u>pril</u> (Altace)

RAM-ih-pril (All-tase)

ANGIOTENSIN II RECEPTOR BLOCKERS (ARBs)

Candesartan (Atacand)
Kan-duh-sar-tan (ah-TUH-kand)

Irbesartan (Avapro)
ihr-buh-sar-tan (ah-VUH-pro)

Irbesartan / Hydrochlorothiazide (Avalide)
lie-SIN-oh-pril / High-droe-klor-oh-THIGH-uh-zide (ah-VUH-lyde)

Losartan (Cozaar)
low-SAR-tan (CO-zar)

> Angiotensin II receptor blockers like **losartan** are often called ARBs and should be learned by the suffix "-sartan." The brand name **Cozaar** looks like it has R-A-A-S backwards (for renin-angiotensin-aldosterone-system) with a "z" replacing the "s."

Losartan / Hydrochlorothiazide (Hyzaar)
lie-SIN-oh-pril / High-droe-klor-oh-THIGH-uh-zide (HIGH-zar)

Olmesartan (Benicar)
Ole-meh-SAR-tan (BEN-eh-car)

> **Olmesartan** is another ARB identified by its "–sartan" stem. The brand name **Benicar** hints that the drug will benefit the cardiac system.

Olmesartan / HCTZ (Benicar HCT)
ole-MEH-sar-tan / High-droe-klor-oh-THIGH-uh-zide (BEN-ih-car)

Telmisartan / HCTZ (Micardis HCT)
tell-MIH-sar-tan / High-droe-klor-oh-THIGH-uh-zide (my-CAR-dis)

Valsartan (Diovan)
val-SAR-tan (DYE-oh-van)

> Identify the generic name **valsartan** by its "–sartan"
> stem. **Diovan** has three of the letters of the generic
> name <u>v</u>als<u>a</u>rt<u>an</u>.

Valsartan / HCTZ (Diovan HCT)
val-SAR-tan / High-droe-klor-oh-THIGH-uh-zide (DYE-oh-van)

ANGIOTENSIN RECEPTOR NEPRILYSIN INHIBITOR (ARNI)

Valsartan / Sacubitril (Entresto)
val-SAR-tan / Sah-CUE-bih-trill (En-TREST-oh)

> **Valsartan** has the "–sartan" stem for an angiotensin
> II receptor blocker, but sacubitril is an angiotensin
> receptor neprilysin inhibitor (ARNI). By the
> blockade of with neprilysin, we prevent natriuretic
> peptide breakdown. The brand name <u>Entr</u>esto is
> meant to convey that you can <u>entr</u>ust the CHF
> patient's care to the medication. The -tril, t-r-i-l
> suffix indicates an endopeptidase inhibitor like
> neprilysin.

V. CALCIUM CHANNEL BLOCKERS (CCBs)

Both calcium channel blocker (CCB) classes, the non-
dihydropyridines and dihydropyridines, are vasodilators.
However, the non-dihydropyridines **diltiazem (Cardizem)**

and **verapamil (Calan)** also affect the heart directly and are antidysrhythmics. **Amlodipine (Norvasc)** and **nifedipine (Procardia)** are two dihydropyridines that only vasodilate.

If a patient needs a calcium channel blocker to prevent uterine contractions, **nifedipine (Procardia)** would be the best choice because it does not suppress the mother's and fetus's hearts as the non-dihydropyridines would.

In our daughters' case, the doctor prescribed low dose **nifedipine** so the calcium channel blockers did not suppress four hearts – my wife's and three unborn daughters'.

NON-DIHYDROPYRIDINES

Diltiazem (Cardizem)
dill-TIE-uh-zem (CAR-deh-zem)

> The "–tiazem" stem identifies **diltiazem** as a non-dihydropyridine. The brand name **Cardizem** adds the first five letters from cardiac to the last three letters of the generic diltiazem.

Verapamil (Calan)
ver-APP-uh-mill (KALE-en)

> One of my students came up with "Vera and Pam are ill and need this calcium blocking cardiac pill," for **verapamil**. Often **verapamil** is associated with constipation. My grandmother, a Navy nurse, used to put a **verapamil** tablet on my grandfather's breakfast cereal spoon. I always thought my grandfather was silently praying before he ate. When I finally asked him why he was so quiet, he said something to the effect of, "I'm deciding whether I want to eat or poop today." The brand

name **Calan** takes three letters from the word
c<u>al</u>cium and two from ch<u>an</u>nel blocker.

DIHYDROPYRIDINES

Amlo<u>dipine</u> (Norvasc)
am-LOW-duh-peen (NOR-vasc)

> Students usually recognize **amlodipine's** "–dipine"
> stem, not only as a <u>dip</u>hydropyri<u>dine</u>, but also as a
> <u>dip in</u> blood pressure. A way to remember the brand
> name **Norvasc** is to think of the "n-o-r" from
> <u>nor</u>malizes and "v-a-s-c" from <u>vasc</u>ulature.

Amlo<u>dipine</u> / Ator<u>vasta</u>tin (Caduet)
am-LOW-duh-peen / uh-TORE-va-stat-in (ka-DU-et)

> This duet of drugs includes a calcium channel
> blocker, **amlodipine**, and **atorvastatin calcium**,
> which is also c-a on the Periodic Table of Elements.

Amlo<u>dipine</u> / Bena<u>zepril</u> (Lotrel)
am-LOW-duh-peen / beh-NAY-zuh-pril (LOW-trell)

> **Benazepril (Lotensin)** becomes **Lotensin HCT**
> when the manufacturer adds **hydrochlorothiazide.**

Amlo<u>dipine</u> / Val<u>sar</u>tan (Exforge)
am-LOW-duh-peen / val-SAR-tan (ECKS-fourge)

Felo<u>dipine</u> (Plendil)
Feh-LOW-dih-peen (PLEN-dill)

Nife<u>dipine</u> (Procardia)
nigh-FED-eh-peen (pro-CARD-e-uh)

Nifedipine is a dihydropyridine with the "–dipine" stem. **Procardia** takes the "p-r-o" from "promotes" and "c-a-r-d-i-a" from "cardiac" so you can remember the brand **Procardia** as promoting cardiac health.

VI. VASODILATOR

Hydralazine (Apresoline)
High-DRAH-luh-zeen (Ah-PRES-uh-leen)

> **Hydralazine** may *cause* angina pectoris.

Isosorbide mononitrate (Imdur)
eye-so-SORE-byde mah-NO-nigh-trate (IM-duhr)

> I grouped **hydralazine** with another vasodilator, **isosorbide dinitrate (Imdur).** The "nitrate" helps you remember this is in the same class as **nitroglycerin.**

Nitroglycerin (Nitrostat)
nigh-trow-GLI-sir-in (NYE-trow-stat)

> "Nitro-"is a World Health Organization (WHO) stem. **Nitroglycerin** converts to nitric oxide, a vasodilator. Make sure the patient sits when he takes the med because it causes significant dizziness. With **Nitrostat**, think "nitrous" from sports cars – the patient and blood pressure drop "stat."

VII. ANTI-ANGINAL

Ranolazine (Ranexa)

ruh-NO-luh-zeen (ruh-NECK-suh)

Ranolazine *treats* angina pectoris.

VIII. Antihyperlipidemics

Medications for elevated cholesterol fall into several categories, including the "statins," which are more properly called the HMG-CoA reductase inhibitors, and the fibric acid derivatives. It's better to recognize statins such as **atorvastatin (Lipitor)** and **rosuvastatin (Crestor)** with the infix + suffix "–vastatin" because **nystatin (Mycostatin)** an antifungal medication contains "statin" in its name.

HMG-CoA reductase inhibitors

Atorvastatin (Lipitor)
uh-TORE-va-stat-in (LIP-eh-tore)

> Students use letters of the HMG-CoA class to memorize potential adverse effects: "H" for hepatotoxicity, "M" for myositis, "G" for gestation (can't use during pregnancy). Brand name **Lipitor** is a lipid gladiator.

Lovastatin (Mevacor)
low-vuh-STAT-in (MEH-vuh-core)

Pravastatin (Pravachol)
prah-vuh-STAT-in (PRAH-vuh-call)

Rosuvastatin (Crestor)
Row-sue-vuh-STAT-in (CRES-tore)

> Like **atorvastatin**, **rosuvastatin** shares the "–vastatin" ending. Remember **Crestor** decreases cholesterol.

339

Simvastatin (Zocor)
sim-vuh-STAT-in (ZO-core)

FIBRIC ACID DERIVATIVES

Fenofibrate (Tricor)
fen-oh-FIE-brate (TRY-core)

> A drug like **fenofibrate** has the obvious stem "–fibrate," a triglyceride lowering fibric acid derivative. **Tricor** lowers triglycerides to help your coronary status.

Gemfibrozil (Lopid)
gem-FIE-broh-zill (LOW-pid)

> The brand names hint at coronary or cholesterol. You can see the "fib" in their fibric acid derivative **gemfibrozil (Lopid).**

BILE ACID SEQUESTRANT

Colesevelam (Welchol)
kow-luh-SEH-vih-lam (WELL-call)

> The bile acid sequestrant **colesevelam (Welchol)** has both a generic and brand name with a hint at cholesterol.

CHOLESTEROL ABSORPTION BLOCKER

Ezetimibe (Zetia)
eh-ZET-uh-mib (ZET-ee-uh)

Ezetimibe (Zetia) is a cholesterol absorption blocker, a different type of drug, and can be combined with an HMG-CoA like **simvastatin (Zocor)** to make **Vytorin**.

Ezetimibe / Simvastatin (Vytorin)
eh-ZET-uh-mib / sim-vuh-STAT-in (VIE-tore-in)

IX. ANTICOAGULANTS AND ANTIPLATELETS

Anticoagulants affect clotting factors to help prevent thrombosis. The injectable anticoagulants **enoxaparin (Lovenox)** or **heparin** and the oral anticoagulant **warfarin (Coumadin)** affect coagulation in slower moving blood vessels like veins. **Dabigatran (Pradaxa)** works as an anticoagulant, but does not require monitoring with blood tests like **warfarin** and **heparin**.

Platelets stop bleeding by creating clots. However, patients with excess cholesterol might have a plaque that makes the clot more likely in a dangerous place. The antiplatelet drugs **aspirin (Ecotrin)** and **clopidogrel (Plavix)** decrease how "sticky" platelets are in high-pressure vessels such as arteries to prevent the clot and ensuing heart attack or stroke.

ANTICOAGULANTS

Enoxaparin (Lovenox)
e-knocks-uh-PEAR-in (LOW-ven-ox)

> **Enoxaparin** and **heparin** share the "–parin" stem because they are related. **Enoxaparin** is more expensive per dose, but patients can use it at home. It's also used as bridge therapy in a patient who is

starting **warfarin** therapy. **Lovenox** is a <u>low</u> molecular weight heparin for deep <u>vein</u> thrombosis prevention.

Heparin
HEP-uh-rin

Heparin and "bleedin'" sort of rhyme to remember its primary adverse effect. A student mentioned the actor Dennis Quaid's twins, who received a double dose of **heparin** that caused bleeding. Sometimes knowing a celebrity with a condition helps memory.

War<u>farin</u> (Coumadin)
WAR-fa-rin (KOO-ma-din)

That the "–parin" stem from the anticoagulants **heparin** and **enoxaparin** and "–farin" stem of **warfarin** are similar. This reminds students they are all anticoagulants. Students associate bleeding with <u>warfare</u>. The INR (<u>i</u>nternational <u>n</u>ormalized <u>r</u>atio), a way of measuring **warfarin's** effectiveness, monitors the patient who is on therapy. "I-N-R" happen to be the last three letters of **warfarin**. A student said that **warfarin** has "far" in it, as in you have to go far to have blood drawn. A way to remember Vitamin K affects **Coumadin** and coagulation is to spell **Coumadin** with a "K" instead of a "C."

Dabi<u>gatran</u> (Pradaxa)
da-bih-GA-tran (pra-DAX-uh)

Memorize **dabigatran's** "–gatran" stem to note the difference between anticoagulants. **Dabigatran** doesn't need INR monitoring like **warfarin** does. Note the last three letters in **dabigatran** as not being "I-N-R."

Rivaroxaban (Xarelto)
riv-uh-RAK-suh-ban (zuh-REL-toe)

The x-a in **rivaroxaban** and **Xarelto** are both meant to indicate the drug's effect on factor 10a as the letter "X" is a ten in Roman numerals. Factor Xa cuts prothrombin to make thrombin and is at the intersection of the intrinsic and extrinsic coagulation pathway.

Apixaban (Eliquis)
uh-PICK-suh-ban (EE-luh-kwus)

ANTIPLATELET

Aspirin / Dipyridamole (Aggrenox)
AS-per-in / die-pir-ih-DUH-mole (AG-ruh-nawks)

Dipyridamole / aspirin (Aggrenox) work together to prevent clots and the brand name can be thought of as "aggregate not."

Clopidogrel (Plavix)
klo-PID-oh-grel (PLA-vix)

Clopidogrel and **aspirin** work similarly leading to a reduced likelihood that platelets will stick together and clot. **Plavix** vexes platelets and keeps the blood thin.

Prasugrel (Effient)
PRAH-Sue-grel (EF-ee-unt)

Effient is the word "efficient" without the "c-i," so may be efficient at thinning platelets.

Ticagrelor (Brilinta)
TIE-cah-greh-lore (brih-LYNN-tuh)

> **Ticagrelor (Brilinta)** has demonstrated superiority to **clopidogrel**. The brand name uses many of the words from brilliant, a British was of saying that's awesome.

X. CARDIAC GLYCOSIDE AND ANTICHOLINERGIC

A cardiac glycoside, such as **digoxin (Lanoxin)**, increases the force of contraction of the heart. We call this a positive inotropic effect. Also an antidysrhythmic, **digoxin** changes the electrochemistry of the heart to prevent dysrhythmias.

Atropine (AtroPen), an anticholinergic, prevents bradycardia, a drop in heart rate. **Atropine** can treat certain cholinergic poisonings.

CARDIAC GLYCOSIDE

Digoxin (Lanoxin)
di-JOCKS-in (la-KNOCKS-in)

> **Digoxin** treats congestive heart failure by increasing the force of the heart's contractions. **Digoxin** is derived from the plant *Digitalis lanata*. In Latin, *Digitalis* means something like hand or "digits," while *lanata* means "wooly" because the actual plant is fuzzy. Therefore, **digoxin** comes from the name *digitalis*, and brand name **Lanoxin** comes from *lanata*. Alternatively, you could remember that **Lanoxin** and **digoxin** keep your heartbeat rockin'.

Atropine (AtroPen)
ah-trow-PEEN (ah-trow-PEN)

> **Atropine** causes anticholinergic (anti = against, cholinergic = of acetylcholine) effects. Anticholinergic effects fall under the broad category of "dry." Use the ABDUCT mnemonic, as in anticholinergics "abduct" water: Anhidrosis, Blurry vision (secondary to dry eyes), Dry mouth, Urinary retention, Constipation, and Tachycardia. This tachycardic side effect therapeutically prevents bradycardia in patients undergoing certain procedures.

> Note: Cholinergic effects would include "wet" effects: sweating, lacrimation (watery eyes), hypersalivation, urinary incontinence, diarrhea, and bradycardia.

XI. ANTIDYSRHYTHMIC

Amiodarone (Cordarone)
ah-MEE-oh-duh-rown (CORE-duh-rone)

> The brand name **Amiodarone (Cordarone)** and the brand and generic share the "arone" lettering. Cardiologists can also use beta-blockers, calcium channel blockers, and **digoxin** as antidysrhythmics.

XII. CARDIODE TO JOY

Cardiode to Joy, sung to the tune of Beethoven's *Ode to Joy*, is a mnemonic that you can sing, hum or just say that attaches many of the common cardio drug endings and classes to their functions.

o-l-o-l-p-r-i-l-and-s-a-r-t-a-n

be-ta-block-er-ace-in-hib-i-tor-and-ARBs-suff-ix-end

as-pir-in-and-clo-pid-o-grel-both-block-plate-lets-round-a-stent

war-fa-rin-and-hep-a-rin-are-both-an-ti-co-ag-u-lants

stat-ins-low-er-chol-est-ter-ol
dig-keeps-your-heart-from-fail-in
ver-a-pa-mil-and-am-lo-di-pine
both-block-cal-cium-chan-nels.

CARDIO DRUG QUIZ (LEVEL 1)

Classify these drugs by placing the corresponding drug class letter next to each medication. Try to underline the stems before you start and think about the brand name and function for each drug.

1. Atorvastatin (Lipitor)
2. Clopidogrel (Plavix)
3. Enalapril (Vasotec)
4. Enoxaparin (Lovenox)
5. Furosemide (Lasix)
6. Hydrochlorothiazide (Microzide)
7. Losartan (Cozaar)
8. Metoprolol (Lopressor)
9. Nifedipine (Procardia)
10. Spironolactone (Aldactone)

Cardio drug classes:

A. ACE inhibitor (ACEI)
B. Alpha blocker
C. Angiotensin receptor blocker (ARB)
D. Anticoagulant
E. Antiplatelet
F. Beta blocker: selective
G. Beta blocker: non-selective
H. CCB – dihydropyridine
I. CCB – non-dihydropyridine
J. Cardiac glycoside
K. Diuretic: Loop
L. Diuretic: Osmotic
M. Diuretic: Potassium sparing
N. Diuretic: Thiazide
O. HMG-CoA reductase inhibitor
P. Vasodilator

CARDIO DRUG QUIZ (LEVEL 2)

Classify these drugs by placing the corresponding drug class letter next to each medication. Try to underline the stems before you start and remember the brand name and function of each drug.

1. Diltiazem
2. Carvedilol
3. Olmesartan
4. Hydrochlorothiazide
5. Doxazosin
6. Amlodipine
7. Nitroglycerin
8. Lisinopril
9. Digoxin
10. Warfarin

Cardio drug classes:

A. ACE inhibitor (ACEI)
B. Alpha blocker
C. Angiotensin receptor blocker (ARB)
D. Anticoagulant
E. Antiplatelet
F. Beta blocker: selective
G. Beta blocker: non-selective
H. CCB – dihydropyridine
I. CCB – non-dihydropyridine
J. Cardiac glycoside
K. Diuretic: Loop
L. Diuretic: Osmotic
M. Diuretic: Potassium sparing
N. Diuretic: Thiazide
O. HMG-CoA reductase inhibitor
P. Vasodilator

PRACTICE EXAM PART 6
CARDIO

QUESTION C1: DIURETIC MECHANISMS OF ACTION

Diuretics have four main points of effect, each with a relatively different degree of diuresis. The medication closest to the glomerulus and most effective in reducing edema would be:

a) Furosemide
b) Hydrochlorothiazide
c) Mannitol
d) Spironolactone

Question C1: Diuretic Mechanisms of Action

Diuretics have four main points of effect, each with a relatively different degree of diuresis. The medication closest to the glomerulus and most effective in reducing edema would be:

 a) Furosemide
 b) Hydrochlorothiazide
 c) Mannitol
 d) Spironolactone

Answer: C. Mannitol (Osmitrol) works in the proximal convoluted tubule, which is the portion of the nephron closest to the glomerulus. The words proximal and proximity, being close to something, are similar. It is the most effective at reducing edema. Furosemide works in the Loop of Henle, Hydrochlorothiazide (HCTZ) in the distal convoluted tubule, and spironolactone in the collecting duct.

QUESTION C2: DIURETIC THERAPEUTICS

While some diuretics have specific indications and others many, often the choice of diuretic comes from the degree of edema or severity of pathophysiologic condition. If a patient had moderate HTN, we would expect _____ as a diuretic choice, and if we were concerned about hypokalemia, we would add _____ .

a) Furosemide, HCTZ
b) HCTZ, Furosemide
c) HCTZ, triamterene
d) Triamterene, HCTZ

Question C2: Diuretic Therapeutics

While some diuretics have specific indications and others many, often the choice of diuretic comes from the degree of edema or severity of pathophysiologic condition. If a patient had moderate HTN, we would expect _____ as a diuretic choice, and if we were concerned about hypokalemia, we would add _____ .

a) Furosemide, HCTZ
b) HCTZ, Furosemide
c) HCTZ, triamterene
d) Triamterene, HCTZ

Answer: C. HCTZ, triamterene (Dyazide). Prescribers give HCTZ for moderate HTN, but it may cause hypokalemia. The potassium-sparing diuretic triamterene works to avoid this problem. We usually don't combine furosemide and HCTZ as the additive effect would increase hypokalemia.

QUESTION C3: DURETIC SIDE EFFECTS

Hyperkalemia and hypokalemia are possible with various diuretics. We would expect which of the following medications to lean toward causing hyperkalemia?

a) Furosemide
b) HCTZ
c) Mannitol
d) Spironolactone

Question C3: Diuretic Side Effects

Hyper and hypokalemia are possible with various diuretics. We would expect which of the following medications to lean toward causing hyperkalemia?

a) Furosemide
b) HCTZ
c) Mannitol
d) Spironolactone

Answer: D. Spironolactone (Aldactone) is a potassium-sparing diuretic that can cause hyperkalemia. Furosemide and HCTZ both release potassium causing hypokalemia.

QUESTION C4: DIURETIC SIDE EFFECTS

Gynecomastia, or breast tissue swelling, is a real concern with which diuretic?

a) Furosemide
b) HCTZ
c) Spironolactone
d) Triamterene

Question C4: Diuretic Side Effects

Gynecomastia, or breast tissue swelling, is a real concern with which diuretic?

a) Furosemide
b) HCTZ
c) Spironolactone
d) Triamterene

Answer: C. Spironolactone can cause hormonal effects and breast tissue swelling.

QUESTION C5: RAAS OVERVEW

The normal effect of angiotensin II release is to cause _____ and _____, helping to increase blood pressure.

a) Vasoconstriction, aldosterone release
b) Vasoconstriction, aldosterone retention
c) Vasodilation, aldosterone release
d) Vasodilation, aldosterone retention

Question C5: RAAS Overview

The normal effect of angiotensin II release is to cause _____ and _____, helping to increase blood pressure.

a) **Vasoconstriction, aldosterone release**
b) Vasoconstriction, aldosterone retention
c) Vasodilation, aldosterone release
d) Vasodilation, aldosterone retention

Answer: A. Vasoconstriction, aldosterone release. Aldosterone affects the kidneys where it causes salt and fluid retention which, in turn, increases blood pressure.

QUESTON C6: ACE INHIBITORS

An ACE inhibitor has the effect of reducing the body's ability to convert angiotensin I into angiotensin II, thus _____ blood pressure. A drug that falls into this category would most likely be _____.

a) Decreasing, lisinopril
b) Decreasing, valsartan
c) Increasing, lisinopril
d) Increasing, valsartan

Question C6: ACE Inhibitors

An ACE inhibitor has the effect of reducing the body's ability to convert angiotensin I into angiotensin II, thus _____ blood pressure. A drug that falls into this category would most likely be _____.

a) Decreasing, lisinopril
b) Decreasing, valsartan
c) Increasing, lisinopril
d) Increasing, valsartan

Answer: A. Decreasing, lisinopril. ACE inhibitors prevent angiotensin II formation, decreasing blood pressure. Lisinopril (Zestril) is an ACE inhibitor, as opposed to losartan, which is an ARB.

QUESTION C7: ANGIOTENSIN RECEPTOR BLOCKERS

An ARB blocks the receptor for _____ and prevents the body from _____ blood vessels thereby decreasing blood pressure.

a) Angiotensin I, vasoconstricting
b) Angiotensin I, vasodilating
c) Angiotensin II, vasoconstricting
d) Angiotensin II, vasodilating

Question C7: Angiotensin Receptor Blockers

An ARB blocks the receptor for _____ and prevents the body from _____ blood vessels thereby decreasing blood pressure.

a) Angiotensin I, vasoconstricting
b) Angiotensin I, vasodilating
c) **Angiotensin II, vasoconstricting**
d) Angiotensin II, vasodilating

Answer: C. Angiotensin II, vasoconstricting. ARBs (like valsartan) block the receptor for angiotensin II preventing its normal vasoconcstriction and increase of blood pressure.

QUESTION C8: CALCIUM CHANNEL BLOCKERS

Sometimes we use technical chemical terms like dihydropyridine and non-dihydropyridine because of a steep difference in the two types of a drug class. Non-Dihydropyridine CCBs affect the _____ and using one _____ make sense when trying to treat dysrhythmias.

a) Heart and vessels, would
b) Heart and vessels, would not
c) Vessels only, would
d) Vessels only, would not

Question C8: Calcium Channel Blockers

Sometimes we use technical chemical terms like dihydropyridine and non-dihydropyridine because of a steep difference in the two types of a drug class. Non-Dihydropyridine CCBs affect the _____ and using one _____ make sense when trying to treat dysrhythmias.

    a) Heart and vessels, would
    b) Heart and vessels, would not
    c) Vessels only, would
    d) Vessels only, would not

Answer: A. Heart and vessels, would. Non-dihydropyridine CCBs like diltiazem (Cardizem) affect the heart and blood vessels; we see their use with dysrhythmias. Dihydropyridines affect blood vessels, and we often use them to treat hypertension.

QUESTION C9: CALCIUM CHANNEL BLOCKERS

A dihydropyridine causes vasodilation just as a non-dihydropyridine CCB does; however, we would expect it's a much better choice for _____. Examples of dihydropyridines include _____ and _____.

a) Dysrhythmias, verapamil and diltiazem
b) Dysrhythmias, verapamil and nifedipine
c) Hypertension, amlodipine and diltiazem
d) Hypertension, amlodipine and nifedipine

Question C9: Calcium Channel Blockers

A dihydropyridine causes vasodilation just as a non-dihydropyridine CCB does; however, we would expect it's a much better choice for _____. Examples of dihydropyridines include _____ and _____.

a) Dysrhythmias, verapamil and diltiazem
b) Dysrhythmias, verapamil and nifedipine
c) Hypertension, amlodipine and diltiazem
d) **Hypertension, amlodipine and nifedipine**

Answer: D. Hypertension, amlodipine and nifedipine. Amlodipine and nifedipine cause vasodilation solely in the blood vessels, making them ideal for treating hypertension. Non-dihydropyridines such as diltiazem and verapamil cause vasodilation in the heart and blood vessels, and are a therapeutic choice for dysrhythmias.

QUESTION C10: BETA-BLOCKERS

Knowing which receptors a medication affects is often fundamental when evaluating a treatment option. When looking at a first-generation beta-blocker, we know that it affects:

a) Beta-1 and beta-2 receptors
b) Beta-1 receptors only
c) Beta-1, beta-2, and alpha-1 receptors
d) Beta-2 receptors only

Question C10: Beta-Blockers

Knowing which receptors a medication affects is often fundamental when evaluating a treatment option. When looking at a first-generation beta-blocker, we know that it affects:

a) **Beta-1 and beta-2 receptors**
b) Beta-1 receptors only
c) Beta-1, beta-2, and alpha-1 receptors
d) Beta-2 receptors only

Answer: A. 1st generation beta-blockers affect both beta-1 and beta-2 receptors affecting the heart and lungs. 2nd generation beta-blockers affect only beta-1 receptors affecting the heart only. 3rd generation beta-blockers block both beta-1 and alpha-1 receptors affecting the heart and blood vessels.

QUESTION C11: BETA-BLOCKER THERAPEUTICS

An asthmatic patient needs to take a beta-blocker for treatment. Which of the following would be a poor choice for this patient?

a) Atenolol
b) Metoprolol succinate
c) Metoprolol tartrate
d) Propranolol

Question C11: Beta-Blocker Therapeutics

An asthmatic patient needs to take a beta-blocker for treatment. Which of the following would be a poor choice for this patient?

a) Atenolol
b) Metoprolol succinate
c) Metoprolol tartrate
d) Propranolol

Answer: D. Propranolol is a 1st-generation non-selective beta-blocker affecting beta-1 and beta-2. The blockade of beta-2 can cause bronchoconstriction, which can be a problem for asthmastics. Atenolol and metoprolol are solely beta-2, so they do not cause bronchoconstriction.

QUESTION C12: BETA-BLOCKER GENERATIONS

Identifying a beta-blocker by generation allows us to better understand what effects it will have on beta, and sometimes alpha, receptors. Identify the 3rd generation beta-blocker below.

a) Atenolol
b) Carvedilol
c) Metoprolol
d) Propranolol

Question C12: Beta-Blocker Generations

Identifying a beta-blocker by generation allows us to better understand what effects it will have on beta, and sometimes alpha, receptors. Identify the 3rd generation beta-blocker below.

a) Atenolol
b) Carvedilol
c) Metoprolol
d) Propranolol

Answer: B. Carvedilol. Propranolol is a 1st generation beta-blocker. Atenolol and metoprolol are 2nd generation beta-blockers. Carvedilol is a 3rd generation beta-blocker.

QUESTION C13: DYSLIPIDEMIA AGENTS

We usually have different names for the same thing in pharmacology. For example, a patient might generally call what he or she takes *a cholesterol medicine*, but as providers we have to be more precise. Which of the following is an HMG-CoA reductase inhibitor?

a) Atorvastatin
b) Gemfibrozil
c) Niacin
d) Omega-3 fatty acids

Question C13: Dyslipidemia Agents

We usually have different names for the same thing in pharmacology. For example, a patient might generally call what he or she takes *a cholesterol medicine*, but as providers we have to be more precise. Which of the following is an HMG-CoA reductase inhibitor?

a) **Atorvastatin**
b) Gemfibrozil
c) Niacin
d) Omega-3 fatty acids

Answer: A. Atorvastatin is an HMG-CoA reductase inhibitor. HMG-CoA is an enzyme responsible for creating cholesterol in hepatocytes, so its inhibition lowers cholesterol levels. Gemfibrozil is a fibrate for hypertriglyceridemia. Omega-3 fatty acids are a good cholesterol supplement. Niacin is a form of vitamin B used in dyslipidemia.

QUESTION C14: HEART FAILURE PATHOLOGY

Heart failure occurs when cardiac output cannot meet oxygen demanded by the tissues, or when it can only meet demand with elevated diastolic blood pressure. The body attempts to compensate for this by _____ preload, afterload, and heart rate; and _____ myocardial contraction strength.

    a) decreasing, increasing
    b) increasing, decreasing
    c) increasing, increasing
    d) decreasing, decreasing

Question C14: Heart Failure Pathology

Heart failure occurs when cardiac output cannot meet oxygen demanded by the tissues, or when it can only meet demand with elevated diastolic blood pressure. The body attempts to compensate for this by _____ preload, afterload, and heart rate; and _____ myocardial contraction strength.

    a) decreasing, increasing
    b) increasing, decreasing
    c) increasing, increasing
    d) decreasing, decreasing

Answer: B. Increasing, decreasing. The body compensates for oxygen demand not being met by increasing preload to put more blood in the ventricle. It compensates by increasing afterload to increase systemic blood pressure. Increasing heart rate keeps blood moving through the tissues. It compensates by decreasing myocardial contraction to decrease oxygen demand. These compensatory mechanisms put a strain on the heart. Heart failure treatment aims to combat these mechanisms.

Question C15: Heart Failure Agents

The first-line therapy for heart failure is the medication class of _____, which decrease preload and afterload through vasodilation. The medication class _____ are similar in action, but they do not have as much clinical-trial data in the setting of heart failure.

a) ACE inhibitors, ARBs
b) ARBs, ACE inhibitors
c) CCBs, Beta-blockers
d) Beta-blockers, CCBs

Question C15: Heart Failure Agents

The first-line therapy for heart failure is the medication
class of _____, which decrease preload and afterload
through vasodilation. The medication class _____ are
similar in action, but they do not have as much clinical-trial
data in the setting of heart failure.

    a) ACE inhibitors, ARBs
    b) ARBs, ACE inhibitors
    c) CCBs, Beta-blockers
    d) Beta-blockers, CCBs

*Answer: A. ACE inhibitors, ARBs. ACE inhibitors are the first
line therapy for HF. ARBs can also be used, but they have less
clinical-trial data supporting them. While we can use beta-
blockers in heart failure, they are not first-line, and act by
decreasing heart rate and thus decreasing oxygen demand in the
myocardium.*

QUESTION C16: ANGINA PECTORIS CLASSIFICATION

There are three main classifications of angina pectoris. Which of the following describes angina that is caused by coronary artery spasm, which leads to decreased oxygen flow to the myocardium?

a) Chronic Stable Angina
b) Variant Angina
c) Unstable Angina
d) Exertional Angina

Question C16: Angina Pectoris Classification

There are three main classifications of angina pectoris. Which of the following describes angina that is caused by coronary artery spasm, which leads to decreased oxygen flow to the myocardium?

a) Chronic Stable Angina
b) **Variant Angina**
c) Unstable Angina
d) Exertional Angina

Answer: B. Variant Angina, or vasospastic angina, comes from coronary artery spasm. Chronic stable (exertional angina) is caused by coronary artery disease (CAD), and it occurs during periods of increased oxygen demand (exertion). Unstable angina is caused by severe CAD which results in a clot or blockage. Unstable angina is unpredictable and constitutes a medical emergency.

QUESTION C17: ANGINA PECTORIS TREATMENT

Some medications are only used in certain kinds of angina. Which of the following medications would not be used for variant (vasospastic) angina?

a) Nitroglycerin
b) Diltiazem
c) Metoprolol
d) Verapamil

Question C17: Angina Pectoris Treatment

Some medications are only used in certain kinds of angina. Which of the following medications would not be used for variant (vasospastic) angina?

a) Nitroglycerin
b) Diltiazem
c) **Metoprolol**
d) Verapamil

Answer: C. Metoprolol. Non-dihydropyridine CCBs such as diltiazem and verapamil are used in both chronic stable and variant angina. Nitroglycerin is also used for both of these kinds of angina.

QUESTION C18: ANTICOAGULANT MEDICATIONS

Both unfractionated and low-molecular weight heparins are used for different reasons. Which of the following is not an advantage of using low-molecular weight heparins such as enoxaparin?

a) It is cheaper than unfractionated heparin
b) No monitoring is required
c) Can be given at home
d) Is equally effective as unfractionated heparin

Question C18: Anticoagulant Medications

Both unfractionated and low-molecular weight heparins are used for different reasons. Which of the following is not an advantage of using low-molecular weight heparins such as enoxaparin?

a) **It is cheaper than unfractionated heparin**
b) No monitoring is required
c) Can be given at home
d) Is equally effective as unfractionated heparin

Answer: A. It is cheaper than unfractionated heparin. Low molecular weight heparin (LMWH) is generally more expensive. However, it requires no monitoring and can be administered at home. LMWH and unfractionated heparin are equally effective.

QUESTION C19: ANTICOAGULANT THERAPEUTICS

A patient reports to your warfarin monitoring clinic after his INR lab came back with a 2.6. What is the next step for adjusting this patient's warfarin therapy?

a) Increase the warfarin dose
b) Decrease the warfarin dose
c) Immediately discontinue warfarin and administer vitamin K
d) No dose change is needed as patient is within INR goal

Question C19: Anticoagulant Therapeutics

A patient reports to your warfarin monitoring clinic after his INR lab came back with a 2.6. What is the next step for adjusting this patient's warfarin therapy?

a) Increase the warfarin dose
b) Decrease the warfarin dose
c) Immediately discontinue warfarin and administer vitamin K
d) No dose change is needed as patient is within INR goal

Answer: D. No dose change is needed as patient is within INR goal. A patient's INR goal is generally between 2.0 and 3.0 for most conditions. If the INR is too high, the warfarin dose should be decreased. If the INR is too low, the dose should be increased. In some situations, with extremely high INRs, the warfarin should be discontinued for the time being and vitamin K should be administered to counteract the warfarin.

QUESTION C20: MYOCARDIAL INFARCTION TREATMENT

A patient comes in currently experiencing an ST-elevated myocardial infarction. Which of the following medications is recommended to reduce platelet aggregation during this event?

a) Morphine
b) Oxygen
c) Nitroglycerin
d) Aspirin

Question C20: Myocardial Infarction Treatment

A patient comes in currently experiencing an ST-elevated myocardial infarction. Which of the following medications is recommended to reduce platelet aggregation during this event?

a) Morphine
b) Oxygen
c) Nitroglycerin
d) Aspirin

Answer: D. Aspirin. Morphine is for MI and pain associated with it. Oxygen is administered to MI patients to increase oxygen flow and decrease infarct size. Nitroglycerin is administered to decrease preload and afterload through vasodilation.

CHAPTER 7 ENDOCRINE / ETC.

I. OTC INSULIN AND EMERGENCY CONTRACEPTION

Most people don't think of insulin as an over-the-counter medication, but a prescription is not required for **regular insulin** or **NPH insulin** (intermediate duration of action) for self-pay patients. Alphabetically "N" comes before "R," but the convention is to put them in order from shortest to longest acting.

Pharmacies refrigerate insulins for stability. Insulins are expensive, so drug stores keep them in the pharmacy refrigerator not only to prevent theft, but so they know that the insulin hasn't left the refrigerator and been exposed to room temperatures. An insulin vial's box has the rectangular shape of a refrigerator to help you remember.

Emergency contraception is a form of birth control used after unprotected sex to keep a patient from getting pregnant. **Levonorgestrel (Plan B)** is a relatively recent introduction. In 1999, it was prescription only, and then it became available behind-the-counter (BTC), but is now available OTC.

Regular insulin (Humulin R)
REG-you-lar IN-su-lin (HUE-myou-lin ARE)

> **Regular insulin** is short acting, but not to be confused with the shortest-acting insulins available, such as **Humalog**. Prescribers can use **regular insulin** when patients need to adjust dosages on a sliding scale. Insulin used to come from a pig

(porcine) or cow (bovine), but now matches human insulin because of molecular engineering. Therefore, the Eli Lilly brand name **Humulin** simply squishes the words <u>hum</u>an and ins<u>ulin</u> together.

NPH insulin (Humulin N)
en-pee-aitch IN-su-lin(HUE-myou-lin EN)

The "N-P-H" in **NPH insulin** stands for <u>n</u>eutral <u>p</u>rotamine <u>H</u>agedorn. The neutral protamine refers to how Hagedorn, the inventor, chemically altered the insulin. The "e-n" pronunciation of the letter "N" sounds a little like "i-n" and can help you remember it's an <u>in</u>termediate acting <u>in</u>sulin.

Levonorgestrel (Plan B One-Step)
LE- vo- nor-JESS-trel (plan-bee won-step)

You can recognize **levonorgestrel** as a progestin hormone product by the "gest" stem. Take it within 72 hours after sexual intercourse. It can cause nausea, so some flat soda might help calm this down. It's now called **Plan B One-Step** because it used to take two steps or two doses to provide this contraception.

I used to work in a college town pharmacy and every Saturday and Sunday morning, I would have a ton of students coming to pick up **Plan B**. Every time, the man drove, and the woman was in the passenger seat. When I told the male student it was fifty bucks for the Plan B, he would invariably look at her, and then pay. One time, however, I overheard her say, "Oh no, you just didn't." Remember the "g-e-s-t" from that "just" that is part of the word **Levonorgestrel**.

II. Diabetes and Insulin

Diabetes mellitus is a condition of chronic excess blood sugar. There are three types: type I, which we previously called juvenile onset diabetes; type II, which we referred to as adult-onset diabetes; and gestational diabetes, a condition where a pregnant woman becomes diabetic. Depending on the condition, there are different drugs that can help lower blood sugar. Almost all oral medications have "gl," or "glu" for "glucose" in their names. Four of these drugs include **metformin (Glucophage), sitagliptin (Januvia), glipizide (Glucotrol)** and **glyburide (DiaBeta)**. I memorized them in alphabetical order of their drug classes: biguanide (**metformin**), dipeptidyl peptidase-4 (DPP-4) (**sitagliptin**), and sulfonylurea (**glipizide** and **glyburide**).

Insulin for diabetes comes from the Latin word insula, which means island. The islets of Langerhans in your pancreas have cells that produce insulin (beta cells), which lowers blood sugar; and cells that produce glucagon (alpha cells), which tells the body to raise blood glucose levels.

There are four major classes of insulin used in treatment:

- *Rapid acting* starts working in 15 minutes and lasts 4 hours, e.g., **insulin lispro (Humalog)**.

- *Short acting* works in 30 minutes and lasts about 6 to 8 hours, e.g., **regular insulin (Humulin R)**.

- *Intermediate duration* **NPH insulin (Humulin N)** works in an hour or two and lasts 14-24 hours.

- *Long duration* **insulin glargine (Lantus, Toujeo)** starts working in an hour and lasts 24 hours.

ORAL ANTI-DIABETICS - BIGUANIDES

Metformin (Glucophage)
met-FOUR-men (GLUE-co-fage)

> One student came up with this mnemonic, "If you
> met four men on **Glucophage**, they are diabetic
> then." Phagocytosis is the process of cell eating. You
> can use the brand name **Glucophage** to think of the
> medication as eating, or "phage-ing" glucose.

Metformin / Glyburide (Glucovance)
met-FOUR-men / GLY-byour-ide (GLEW-co-vance)

> Manufacturers combine the biguanide **metformin
> (Glucophage)** with the sulfonylurea **glyburide
> (DiaBeta)** to make **Glucovance** – an advance in
> glucose lowering.

ORAL ANTI-DIABETICS – DPP-4 INHIBITORS

Linagliptin (Tradjenta)
lin-uh-GLIP-tuhn (truh-JEN-tuh)

Saxagliptin (Onglyza)
sak-suh-GLIP-tuhn (awn-GLI-zuh)

> Patients refer to DPP-4 inhibitors **linagliptin
> (Tradjenta)** and **saxagliptin (Onglyza)** by their stem
> "-gliptin."

Sitagliptin (Januvia)
sit-uh-GLIP-tin (ja-NEW-vee-uh)

> Although the "-gliptin" stem helps us recognize
> **sitagliptin** as an anti-diabetic, students associate the

sugar you might put in "Lipton" iced tea with **sitagliptin**. The brand name **Januvia** ends in "v-i-a" and is similar to "d-i-a" from dia̲betes.

MEGLITINIDES (GLINIDES)

Repaglinide̲ (Prandin)
rih-PAH-glih-nide (PRAN-din)

> The meglitinide **repaglinide̲ (Prandin),** as a "-glinide."

ORAL ANTI-DIABETICS – SULFONYLUREAS 2ND-GENERATION

Glipizide̲ (Glucotrol)
GLIP-eh-zide (GLUE-co-trawl)

> The "gli-" stem in **glipizide̲** and **glimepiride̲** next indicate an antihyperglycemic medication. The brand name **Glucotrol** alludes to the contr̲ol of blood gluco̲se in diabetics.

Glimepiride̲ (Amaryl)
glih-MEH-puh-ride (AM-uh-rill)

Glyburide̲ (DiaBeta)
GLY-byour-ide (die-uh-BAY-ta)

> The "gly-" stem in **glyburide̲** is archaic and has been replaced in new medicines by the stem "gli-." The brand name **DiaBeta** combines the "d-i-a" from dia̲betic, and the "B-e-t-a" from the Beta̲ cells, which release insulin.

THIAZOLIDINEDIONES (GLITAZONES)

Pioglitazone (Actos)
pie-uh-GLIH-tuh-zone (AK-toes)

Rosiglitazone (Avandia)
row-suh- GLIH-tuh-zone (uh-van-DEE-uh)

INCRETIN MIMETICS

Exenatide (Byetta)
eck-ZEN-uh-tide (BUY-eh-tuh)

>An injectable antidiabetic.

Liraglutide (Victoza)
lih-RAH-glue-tide (VIK-toe-zuh)

>Another injectable.

HYPOGLYCEMIA

Glucagon (GlucaGen)
GLUE-ca-gone (glue-ca-JEN)

>Remember the generic with, "I use **glucagon** when the glucose is gone." **GlucaGen,** the brand name, generates glucose when a patient is hypoglycemic.

RX INSULIN

Insulin aspart (Novolog)
IN-su-lin AS-part (NO-vuh-lawh)

Insulin aspart (Novolog) is another insulin analog.

Insulin lispro (Humalog)
IN-su-lin LICE-pro (HUE-muh-lawg)

> **Insulin glargine** would precede **insulin lispro** alphabetically, but the convention is to list the medications shorter acting to longer acting. I use my Spanish language to help memorize that **insulin lispro** is rapid acting. When I was in Mexico on a zip line, the person in the first tower would say, "Listo, listo," meaning "You ready, I'm ready." Then I would fly fast down that zip cord. **Humalog** is a human insulin analog. I always pictured a log floating down rapids fast to remember **Humalog** is a rapid acting insulin.

Insulin detemir (Levemir)
IN-su-lin DEH-tuh-meer (LEH-vuh-meer)

> **Insulin detemir (Levemir)** is a long-acting insulin like **Lantus**.

Insulin glargine (Lantus, Toujeo)
IN-su-lin GLAR-Jean (LAN-tuss, TWO-jzeh-oh)

> With **insulin glargine**, I think of glaring and lurking, someone who is *slowly* creeping around. One student came up with "**Lantus** lasts all day long, take it at night, and your life will be prolonged." I've also heard "lazy **Lantus**" used to help remember it's a 24-hour drug.

III. THYROID HORMONES

Thyroid hormone stimulates the heart, metabolism, and helps with growth. A hyperthyroid patient's body uses energy too quickly because of the extra thyroid hormone in circulation.

This patient can use **propylthiouracil (PTU)** to reduce the effects of the thyroid hormone. Hypothyroid patients need extra thyroid hormone, such as **levothyroxine (Synthroid)**, for replacement.

HYPOTHYROIDISM

Levothyroxine (Synthroid)
Lee-vo-thigh-ROCKS-een (SIN-throyd)

> The generic name **levothyroxine** has the "thyro" from thyroid in the name; you just have to remember it's for supplementation. The brand name **Synthroid** combines the words synthetic and thyroid.

HYPERTHYROIDISM

Propylthiouracil (PTU)
pro-pill-thigh-oh-YOUR-uh-sill (pee-tee-you)

> **PTU** takes "p" from propyl, "t" from "thio," and "u" from uracil in the generic **propylthiouracil**. Although "thio" means there is a sulfur atom in the molecule, you can think of it as thyroid lowering.

IV. Hormones and contraception

Testosterone is an androgen steroid hormone that naturally comes from the male testes. As a medication, prescribers use it to supplement conditions of low testosterone.

Pharmaceutical birth control, commonly known as "the pill," traditionally came from a combined oral contraceptive pill (COCP) that has a combination of an estrogen and a progestin. There are many variations of "the pill" including **Loestrin 24 Fe.** The Fe stands for <u>fe</u>rrous, or iron, on the periodic table. The tri-phasic birth controls, such as **Tri-Sprintec**, have three different doses of an estrogen and progestin, taken variously throughout the month to mimic the body's naturally changing hormone levels. Two novel birth control delivery methods include a vaginally inserted ring **(NuvaRing)** and a transdermal patch **(OrthoEvra).**

Testosterone

Testo<u>ster</u>one (AndroGel)
Tess-TOSS-ter-own (ANN-droh GEL)

> Most people know the steroid hormone **testosterone**, but note the stem for a steroid is "ster." "<u>Andro</u>" is the Greek prefix for male and <u>gel</u> is the vehicle in **AndroGel**, indicating it's a "gel" for a "male."

Estrogens and / or Progestins

In the following few meds you'll see the estrogen stem "estr, e-s-t-r" and progestin stem "-gest, g-e-s-t" which are sometimes easily confused.

Estradiol (Estrace, Estraderm)
es-truh-DIE-aw (ES-trays, ES-truh-derm)

> The Estr, e-s-t-r stem is for estrogen. The Estrace
> name is a pill while the Estraderm is a patch with
> the "derm" for dermatologic.

Conjugated estrogens (Premarin)
KAHN-juh-ga-tuhd EH-stroe-jens (PREH-muh-rin)

> The **Premarin** brand name is short for pregnant
> mare's urine, full of estrogens.

Conjugated estrogens / Medroxyprogesterone (PremPro/PremPhase)
KAHN-juh-ga-tuhd EH-stroe-jens / meh-DROCK-see-proh-jes-ter-own (PREM-pro / PREM-faze)

> **PremPro** is a single tablet that a patient takes once a
> day. **PremPhase** has dosing in two phases, one for
> fourteen days, another with both conjugated
> estrogens and medroxyprogesterone for the other 14
> days.

Progesterone (Prometrium)
proh-JES-ter-own (PRO-me-tree-um)

> **Prometrium** is not just "pro, p-r-o" for progesterone,
> but also a hint that it is pro, or good for the
> endometrium. Prometrium prevents endometrial
> hyperplasia and secondary amenorrhea symptoms.

Medroxyprogesterone (Provera)
meh-DROCK-see-proh-jes-ter-own (PROH-ver-uh)

> **Provera** hints at preventing abnormal uterine
> bleeding or provide treatment for absent or irregular

periods. **Provera**, prevent, and provide all shore letters together.

CONTRACEPTION – COMBINED ORAL CONTRACEPTIVES

Norethindrone / ethinyl estradiol / ferrous fumarate (Loestrin 24 Fe)
Nor-eth-IN-drone / ETH-in-ill es-tra-DYE-all (Low-ES-trin EF-ee Twen-TEE fore)

> It's important to first memorize the estrogen stem "estr-" and progestin stem "-gest-." Then I got a little rhyme crazy with the contraceptive brand name mnemonics. One rhyme goes: "**Loestrin 24 Fe** reduces the length of menstruation, with iron supplementation, to prevent an anemic situation."

Norgestimate / ethinyl estradiol (Tri-Sprintec)
Nor-JESS-teh-mate / ETH-in-ill es-tra-DYE-all"

> For most hormone-based contraceptives, it's important to note both the estrogen stem "estr-"and progestin stem "-gest-." And here's another rhyme: "**Tri-Sprintec** is triphasic, take three different doses, in seven-day spaces."

CONTRACEPTION – PATCH

Norelgestromin / ethinyl estradiol (Xulane)
Nor-el-JESS-tro-min / ETH-in-ill es-tra-DYE-all (OR-thoe EV-rah)

> One student thought of the "Norel" in **norelgestromin** as "not oral" to remember this is a patch. Another rhyme highlights the places a woman should place the patch and length of time to

leave it there: **"Xulane** is a patch, put it on your arm, your abs, your buttock or back, and then take it off a week after that."

CONTRACEPTION – RING

Etonogestrel / ethinyl estradiol (NuvaRing)
Et-oh-no-JESS-trel / ETH-in-ill es-tra-DYE-all"
(NEW-va-ring)

> A student thought of the "Etono" in **etonogestrel** as "Eat, oh no" to remember it's not an oral tablet. A final rhyme and then I promise, no more: "**NuvaRing** is one way to keep the stork away before you are ready for parenting a bay-bay" (By the way, just as an aside, there is no time when you are actually ready for parenting.)

V. OVERACTIVE BLADDER, URINARY RETENTION, ERECTILE DYSFUNCTION, BENIGN PROSTATIC HYPERPLASIA

Frequently the words incontinence, urinary retention, impotence, and benign prostatic hyperplasia are confused:

- **Overactive bladder (OAB) (incontinence)** is an inability to retain urine due to overactive bladder.
- **Urinary retention** is a difficulty in urination.
- **Erectile dysfunction (ED) (impotence)** is the inability to achieve or maintain an erection.
- **Benign prostatic hyperplasia (BPH)** is a benign (not harmful) prostate growth or increase in size.

We try not to use the terms "incontinence" or "impotence" because of the harshness of the words.

OVERACTIVE BLADDER

Oxybutynin (Ditropan, Oxytrol OTC)
ox-e-BYOU-tin-in (DIH-trow-pan)

> One student remembered **oxybutynin** as keepin' the urin' in. Both **Ditropan** and **Oxytrol** have the "t-r-o" from control for controlling an overactive bladder.

Darifenacin (Enablex)
dar-ih-FEN-uh-sin (en-AA-blecks)

> **Darifenacin (Enablex)** and **solifenacin (VESIcare)** have the same "–fenacin" stem. Both work for overactive bladder (OAB). The **Enablex** brand name hints at "enabling" the patient to "exit" the house when the OAB might have kept them in.

Solifenacin (VESIcare)
sol-ih-FEN-uh-sin (VEH-si-care)

> **Solifenacin** is given once daily, so thinking about it as "slow-fenacin" helps in remembering this point. Also, **solifenacin** solves the problem of urine that needs to be "fenced in." **VESIcare** contains *vesica,* which means "bladder" in Latin.

Tolterodine (Detrol)
toll-TER-oh-dean (DEH-trawl)

> The generic name **tolterodine** has the "t-r-o" from control in the name as well. **Detrol** helps control the detrusor muscle, keeping urine in.

URINARY RETENTION

Bethanechol (Urecholine)

beh-THAN-uh-call (yur-eh-CO-lean)

> The "chol" in **bethanechol** helps you remember it's
> cholinergic. While anticholinergics are dry,
> cholinergics do the opposite and make things wet.
> This drug assists the bladder muscles in expelling
> urine. The brand name **Urecholine** alludes to how it
> affects urination through cholinergic effects.

ERECTILE DYSFUNCTION (PDE-5 INHIBITORS)

Sildenafil (Viagra)
sill-DEN-uh-fill (vie-AG-rah)

> There is a scene with Jack Nicholson in the movie
> *Something's Gotta Give* that reminds us **sildenafil**
> shouldn't be used with nitrates like **nitroglycerin**.
> **Viagra** brings viable growth – an erection.

Vardenafil (Levitra)
var-DEN-uh-fill (leh-VEE-truh)

> **Vardenafil (Levitra)** seems to have the same "-den-"
> infix as **sildenafil** (**Viagra**). To levitate is to rise
> above the ground, so the brand **Levitra** hints at the
> rising erection.

Tadalafil (Cialis)
ta-DAL-uh-fill (see-AL-is)

> **Cialis** is the weekend pill because it, unlike
> **sildenafil**, lasts the weekend, as it has a long half-
> life. I asked some students about how they
> remembered **tadalafil** and I'm hesitant to share their
> mnemonic. One said you just think "ta-dah" as in
> "surprise." I stopped them before they started on to

how they remember the "fil" part of the generic name. **Cialis** is the dual bathtub commercials drug.

BPH – ALPHA BLOCKER

Tamsulosin (Flomax)
tam-syoo-LOW-sin (FLOW-Max)

> **Flomax** allows for <u>max</u>imum urinary <u>flow</u>. The "osin" ending is not an actual stem, but a way to connect **tamsulosin** and **alfuzosin** as being similar.

Alfuzosin (Uroxatral)
al-fyoo-ZOH-sin (YUR-ox-uh-trall)

> With BPH, there is sometimes difficulty with urine control and I think the brand **Uroxatral** sounds a little like "<u>U</u>rine con<u>trol</u>."

BPH – 5-ALPHA-REDUCTASE INHIBITOR

Dutasteride (Avodart)
due-TAS-ter-ide (AH-vo-dart)

> Use the "–steride" stem to recognize the 5-alpha-reductase inhibitors like **dutasteride**. The "ster" for steroid helps you remember it's for men (and prostate).

Finasteride (Proscar, Propecia)
fin-AS-ter-ide" (PRO-scar, pro-PEE-shuh)

> To connect the brand name **Proscar** to the generic **finasteride**, a professor told me of a student who used the phrase "That <u>pro's car</u> is the <u>finest ride</u>." **Proscar** is for <u>pros</u>tate **car**e. **Finasteride's** other

brand name, **Propecia**, alludes to hair growth and is
to reverse al<u>opecia</u> (hair loss).

ENDOCRINE / MISC. DRUG QUIZ (LEVEL 1)

Classify these drugs by placing the corresponding drug class letter next to each medication. Try to underline the stems before you start and think about the brand name and function of each drug.

1. Glipizide (Glucotrol)
2. Glucagon (GlucaGen)
3. Glyburide (DiaBeta)
4. Insulin glargine (Lantus)
5. Levothyroxine (Synthroid)
6. Metformin (Glucophage)
7. Propylthiouracil (PTU)
8. Regular insulin (Humulin R)
9. Solifenacin (VESIcare)
10. Sildenafil (Viagra)

Endocrine system drug classes:

A. Anti-diabetic
B. BPH - 5-alpha-reductase inhibitor
C. BPH - alpha blocker
D. Contraception – COCP triphasic
E. Contraception – COCP with iron
F. Contraception – patch
G. Contraception – ring
H. For hypoglycemia
I. For hypothyroidism
J. For hyperthyroidism
K. Erectile dysfunction
L. OAB
M. Insulin – long acting
N. Insulin – short acting
O. Urinary retention

ENDOCRINE / MISC. DRUG QUIZ (LEVEL 2)

Classify these drugs by placing the corresponding drug class letter next to each medication. Try to underline the stems before you start and remember the brand name and function of each drug.

1. Dutasteride
2. Tamsulosin
3. Tolterodine
4. Tadalafil
5. Norethindrone / ethinyl estradiol / Fe
6. Norelgestromin / ethinyl estradiol
7. Oxybutynin
8. Bethanechol
9. Sildenafil
10. Finasteride

Endocrine system drug classes:

A. Anti-diabetic
B. BPH - 5-alpha-reductase inhibitor
C. BPH - alpha blocker
D. Contraception – COCP triphasic
E. Contraception – COCP with iron
F. Contraception – patch
G. Contraception – ring
H. For hypoglycemia
I. For hypothyroidism
J. For hyperthyroidism
K. Erectile dysfunction
L. OAB
M. Insulin – long acting
N. Insulin – short acting
O. Urinary retention

PRACTICE EXAM PART 7
ENDOCRINE, ETC.

QUESTION E1: DIABETES PATHOLOGY

Knowing the effects of glucagon and insulin are critical to understanding how the body regulates blood sugar. When the body releases glucagon, we expect a _____ in blood sugar. When the body releases insulin, this causes a _____ in blood sugar.

a) Reduction, reduction
b) Reduction, rise
c) Rise, reduction
d) Rise, rise

Question E1: Diabetes Pathology

Knowing the effects of glucagon and insulin are critical to understanding how the body regulates blood sugar. When the body releases glucagon, we expect a _____ in blood sugar. When the body releases insulin, this causes a _____ in blood sugar.

a) Reduction, reduction
b) Reduction, rise
c) **Rise, reduction**
d) Rise, rise

Answer: C. Rise, reduction. The liver releases glucagon as a response to low blood sugar. The pancreas releases insulin to help store glucose reducing blood levels.

QUESTION E2: DIABETES SYMPTOMATOLOGY

Diabetics can experience excessive thirst known as
_____. And we might also see _____ which is
excessive urination.

    a) Polydipsia, polyuria
    b) Polyuria, polydipsia
    c) Xerostomia, ketonuria
    d) Xerostomia, polyuria

Question E2: Diabetes Symptomatology

Diabetics can experience excessive thirst known as
_____. And we might also see _____ which is
excessive urination.

    a) Polydipsia, polyuria
    b) Polyuria, polydipsia
    c) Xerostomia, ketonuria
    d) Xerostomia, polyuria

*Answer: A. Polydipsia is the term for excessive thirst and
polyuria means excessive urination. Ketonuria indicates ketones,
a possible sign of diabetic ketoacidosis. Xerostomia describes dry
mouth, a common side effect of some antidepressants.*

QUESTION E3: DIABETES MEDICATIONS

The biguanide antidiabetic medication is notorious for its GI effects. Often, it's better to start low and go slowly, otherwise the effects will make a patient discontinue a very good drug. Which of the following is that biguanide?

a) Glipizide
b) Glucagon
c) Glyburide
d) Metformin

Question E3: Diabetes Medications

The biguanide antidiabetic medication is notorious for its GI effects. Often, it's better to start low and go slowly, otherwise the effects will make a patient discontinue a very good drug. Which of the following is that biguanide?

   a) Glipizide
   b) Glucagon
   c) Glyburide
   d) Metformin

Answer: D. Metformin (Glucophage) is a biguanide medication, and it is a first line treatment for Type II and gestational diabetes. Glipizide (Glucotrol) and glyburide (DiaBeta) are sulfonylureas and glucagon (GlucaGen) elevates blood sugar.

QUESTION E4: INSULIN MEDICATIONS

We're especially interested in how quickly or slowly an insulin works. When considering the most rapid-acting insulin we think of:

a) Insulin glargine
b) Insulin lispro
c) NPH insulin
d) Regular insulin

Question E4: Insulin Medications

We're especially interested in how quickly or slowly an insulin works. When considering the most rapid-acting insulin we think of:

a) Insulin glargine
b) Insulin lispro
c) NPH insulin
d) Regular insulin

Answer: B. Insulin lispro is the most rapid-acting insulin. Regular insulin is short-acting, NPH insulin is intermediate-acting, and insulin glargine is long-acting.

QUESTION E5: INSULIN MEDICATIONS

When looking for an insulin that can cover most of the day, we look to which drug?

a) Insulin glargine
b) Insulin lispro
c) NPH insulin
d) Regular insulin

Question E5: Insulin Medications

When looking for an insulin that can cover most of the day, we look to which drug?

a) Insulin glargine
b) Insulin lispro
c) NPH insulin
d) Regular insulin

Answer: A. Insulin glargine (Lantus) is the longest-acting insulin working for 24 hours. While NPH insulin (Humulin N) lasts for a while, it only lasts around 8-12 hours, so it cannot cover most of the day.

QUESTION E6: DIABETES MEDICATIONS

All of the following have an effect of increasing insulin release or promoting insulin secretion except:

a) Glipizide
b) Glyburide
c) Metformin
d) Sitagliptin

Question E6: Diabetes Medications

All of the following have an effect of increasing insulin release or promoting insulin secretion except:

    a) Glipizide
    b) Glyburide
    c) Metformin
    d) Sitagliptin

Answer: C. Metformin (Glucophage), a biguanide, works by stopping intestinal absorption of glucose, stopping the liver from making glucose, and promoting insulin sensitivity. Sulfonylureas such as glipizide (Glucotrol), glyburide (DiaBeta) and DPP4 inhibitors like sitagliptin (Januvia) all work by stimulating insulin secretion from the pancreas. [Do not repeat slide]

QUESTION E7: DIABETES THERAPEUTICS

Sometimes a **patient's** other diseases dictate our direction
with a certain diabetic therapy. This medication is
something we tend to avoid with kidney disease because of
our concern about lactic acidosis.

a) Metformin
b) Regular insulin
c) Glyburide
d) Sitagliptin

Question E7: Diabetes Therapeutics

Sometimes a **patient's** other diseases dictate our direction with a certain diabetic therapy. This medication is something we tend to avoid with kidney disease because of our concern about lactic acidosis.

a) **Metformin**
b) Regular insulin
c) Glyburide
d) Sitagliptin

Answer: A. Metformin. The body excretes metformin (Glucophage) solely by the kidney. When the kidneys are not functioning fully, metformin can build up and lead to lactic acidosis. None of the other options have this issue. [Do not repeat slide]

QUESTION E8: DIABETES THERAPEUTICS

We know beta blockers can affect heart rate, but in diabetes we're concerned that a beta blocker will mask the _____ a patient feels when he or she is _____ ?

a) Tachycardia, hypoglycemic
b) Tachycardia, hyperglycemic
c) Bradycardia, hypoglycemic
d) Bradycardia, hyperglycemic

Question E8: Diabetes Therapeutics

We know beta blockers can affect heart rate, but in diabetes we're concerned that a beta blocker will mask the _____ a patient feels when he or she is _____?

a) **Tachycardia, hypoglycemic**
b) Tachycardia, hyperglycemic
c) Bradycardia, hypoglycemic
d) Bradycardia, hyperglycemic

Answer: A. Tachycardia, hypoglycemic. Hypoglycemia can cause a light-headedness, dizziness, and increased heart rate (tachycardia). We worry beta-blockers will mask this hypoglycemia symptom.

QUESTION E9: DIABETES MONITORING

When a provider wants to know the average of the patient's blood sugars over the past three months, he or she would look to the patient's:

a) Fasting blood glucose
b) Glucometer memory
c) Glycosylated hemoglobin A1c
d) Postprandial blood glucose

Question E9: Diabetes Monitoring

When a provider wants to know the average of the patient's blood sugars over the past three months, he or she would look to the patient's:

a) Fasting blood glucose
b) Glucometer memory
c) **Glycosylated hemoglobin A1c**
d) Postprandial blood glucose

Answer: C. Glycosylated hemoglobin A1C. Fasting blood glucose tests let us know a patient's current blood sugar, but glycosylated hemoglobin A1C tests for the blood cells that have glucose attached. The cells last for around 3 months, and this test gives us a good average of that time.

QUESTION E10: THYROID DISORDER SYMPTOMATOLOGY

Hyperthyroidism would most likely present with all of the following factors except:

a) Nervousness
b) Tremors
c) Weight gain
d) Anorexia

Question E10: Thyroid Disorder Symptomatology

Hyperthyroidism would most likely present with all of the following factors except:

a) Nervousness
b) Tremors
c) **Weight gain**
d) Anorexia

Answer: C. Weight gain. Hypothyroidism presents with fatigue, weight gain, shakiness, and chills. Hyperthyroidism symptoms include insomnia, anorexia, nervousness, tremors, and sweating.

QUESTION E11: THYROID DISORDER THERAPEUTICS

When treating hyperthyroidism, we expect a patient to have a _____ and use _____ as a possible treatment.

a) High TSH, levothyroxine
b) High TSH, propylthiouracil
c) Low TSH, levothyroxine
d) Low TSH, propylthiouracil

Question E11: Thyroid Disorder Therapeutics

When treating hyperthyroidism, we expect a patient to have a _____ and use _____ as a possible treatment.

a) High TSH, levothyroxine
b) High TSH, propylthiouracil
c) Low TSH, levothyroxine
d) Low TSH, propylthiouracil

Answer: D. Low TSH, propylthiouracil. A hyperthyroid patient already has significant thyroid hormone so thyroid stimulating hormone (TSH) is low. Propylthiouracil reduces thyroid hormone levels; levothyroxine raises them.

QUESTION E12: THYROID DISORDER MEDICATIONS

Levothyroxine is used for hypothyroidism, and it acts as a replacement for which hormone?

a) Thyroxine
b) Thyroid-stimulating hormone
c) Progesterone
d) Estrogen

Question E12: Thyroid Disorder Medications

Levothyroxine is used for hypothyroidism, and it acts as a replacement for which hormone?

a) **Thyroxine**
b) Thyroid-stimulating hormone
c) Progesterone
d) Estrogen

Answer: A. Thyroxine. Levothyroxine (Synthroid) is a synthetic version of thyroxine. TSH would already be elevated in hypothyroidism. Estrogen and progesterone are involved in other aspects of hormonal balance.

QUESTION E13: TESTOSTERONE COUNSELING

A patient asks about topical testosterone supplementation. Which of the following should not be a part of your counseling?

a) Acne, prostate enlargement, and gynecomastia are possible.
b) Androgel is synthetic, but otherwise identical to natural testosterone.
c) Leave application areas uncovered.
d) Androgel is for low testosterone levels.

Question E13: Testosterone Counseling

A patient asks about topical testosterone supplementation. Which of the following should not be a part of your counseling?

    a) Acne, prostate enlargement, and gynecomastia are possible.
    b) Androgel is synthetic, but otherwise identical to natural testosterone.
    c) Leave application areas uncovered.
    d) Androgel is for low testosterone levels.

Answer: C. Leave application areas uncovered. Cover application areas to avoid transferring to children. The other options are correct.

QUESTION E14: BIRTH CONTROL NOMENCLATURE

A patient is looking for the estrogen component in her birth control combination; we would expect these four letters to identify that component.

a) Este
b) Estr
c) Gest
d) Ster

Question E14: Birth Control Nomenclature

A patient is looking for the estrogen component in her birth control combination; we would expect these four letters to identify that component.

- a) Este
- **b) Estr**
- c) Gest
- d) Ster

Answer: B. Estr. The stem estr- indicates estrogen. The stem -gest- indicates progesterone, -ster- indicates steroid, and este is not a stem.

QUESTION E15: BIRTH CONTROL FORMULATION

Norgestimate/ethinyl estradiol (Tri-Sprintec) administers 3 different hormone levels over the cycle starting with more estrogen at the beginning and ending with more progesterone. Why?

a) The levels oppose the natural menstruation cycle, preventing pregnancy
b) It provides hormone levels similar to the natural menstruation
c) A stronger starting dose reduces side effects
d) The administration reduces menstruation length

Question E15: Birth Control Formulation

Norgestimate/ethinyl estradiol as Tri-Sprintec administers 3 different hormone levels over the cycle starting with more estrogen at the beginning and ending with more progesterone. Why?

a) The levels oppose the natural menstruation cycle, preventing pregnancy
b) It provides hormone levels similar to the natural menstruation
c) A stronger starting dose reduces side effects
d) The administration reduces menstruation length

Answer: B. It provides hormone levels similar to the natural menstruation. Tri-Sprintec is formulated with 3 hormone levels to better mimic the natural hormone levels of the natural cycle of menstruation.

QUESTION E16: OVERACTIVE BLADDER

Which of the following is not an antimuscarinic medication for overactive bladder (OAB) treatment?

a) Tolterodine
b) Bethanechol
c) Solifenacin
d) Oxybutynin

Question E16: Overactive Bladder

Which of the following is not an antimuscarinic medication for overactive bladder (OAB) treatment?

a) Tolterodine
b) Bethanechol
c) Solifenacin
d) Oxybutynin

Answer: B. Bethanechol (Urecholine) is a cholinergic agent for urinary retention that increases bladder smooth-muscle contractility; in other words, it makes overactive bladder worse. Tolterodine (Detrol), solifenacin (VESIcare), and oxybutynin (Ditropan) are all antimuscarinic agents for overactive bladder. They relax the bladder's smooth-muscle wall to better fill before emptying.

QUESTION E17: BPH MEDICATIONS

Benign prostatic hyperplasia (BPH) is a condition of an enlarged prostate that often inhibits urine flow. Treatment can come by increasing the urethra diameter or shrinking the prostate. Which medication shrinks the prostate?

a) Dutasteride
b) Tamsulosin
c) Sildenafil
d) Alfuzosin

Question E17: BPH Medications

Benign prostatic hyperplasia (BPH) is a condition of an enlarged prostate that often inhibits urine flow. Treatment can come by increasing the urethra diameter or shrinking the prostate. Which medication shrinks the prostate?

a) **Dutasteride**
b) Tamsulosin
c) Sildenafil
d) Alfuzosin

Answer: A. Dutasteride (Avodart) works on BPH by shrinking the prostate. Sildenafil (Viagra) helps erectile dysfunction and BPH symptoms. Tamsulosin (Flomax) and alfuzosin (Uroxatral) both work in BPH by increasing the urethra diameter.

QUESTION E18: BPH MEDICATION ONSET OF ACTION

When a patient needs relatively quick relief of BPH symptoms, we know that it will likely fall on a medication like:

a) Dutasteride
b) Finasteride
c) Propranolol
d) Tamsulosin

Question E18: BPH Medication Onset of Action

When a patient needs relatively quick relief of BPH symptoms, we know that it will likely fall on a medication like:

a) Dutasteride
b) Finasteride
c) Propranolol
d) Tamsulosin

Answer: D. Tamsulosin, an alpha blocker, works by directly relaxing the prostate and increasing the urethra diameter. This process is much faster than the 5-alpha reductase inhibitor-decreasing hormone production to shrink the prostate. Propranolol is a beta blocker, rather than an alpha blocker, that would not help this patient.

QUESTION E19: BPH MEDICATION CLASSES

When treating BPH, often the early use of an alpha blocker will precede the longer time it takes for a 5-alpha reductase inhibitor to work. Which pairing represents an alpha blocker and then a 5-alpha reductase inhibitor?

a) Alfuzosin, sildenafil
b) Alfuzosin, tamsulosin
c) Dutasteride, finasteride
d) Tamsulosin, dutasteride

Question E19: BPH Medication Classes

When treating BPH, often the early use of an alpha blocker will precede the longer time it takes for a 5-alpha reductase inhibitor to work. Which pairing represents an alpha-blocker and then a 5-alpha reductase inhibitor?

a) Alfuzosin, sildenafil
b) Alfuzosin, tamsulosin
c) Dutasteride, finasteride
d) Tamsulosin, dutasteride

Answer: D. Tamsulosin is an alpha-blocker and dutasteride is a 5-alpha reductase inhibitor. While alfuzosin is an alpha blocker as well, the other choices pair it with a PDE-5 or second alpha blocker which we would not do therapeutically.

QUESTION E20: ERECTILE DYSFUNCTION

When treating erectile dysfunction, we expect to see a medication like _____ which represents the _____ class of drugs.

a) Dutasteride, 5-alpha reductase inhibitors
b) Dutasteride, PDE-5
c) Sildenafil, 5-alpha reductase inhibitors
d) Sildenafil, PDE-5

Question E20: Erectile Dysfunction

When treating erectile dysfunction, we expect to see a medication like _____ which represents the _____ class of drugs.

a) Dutasteride, 5-alpha reductase inhibitors
b) Dutasteride, PDE-5
c) Sildenafil, 5-alpha reductase inhibitors
d) Sildenafil, PDE-5

Answer: D. Sildenafil is a phosphodiesterase five (PDE-5) inhibitor for erectile dysfunction. Dutasteride is a 5-alpha reductase inhibitor for BPH.

Memorizing Pharmacology

CHAPTER 8 A FEW PRACTICE QUESTIONS ON SUPPLEMENTS

With supplements and herbals, it's just easiest if I give you a mnemonic to remember why someone would most likely reason someone would take them.

I'm not saying any of these supplments actually work for the condition, I'm just saying this is what customers come in for and why.

You can use the EPICARDIUM mnemonic. While I get the epicardium is the outer surface of the heart membrane, it just seemed appropriate to connect heart and herbals.

MNEMONIC – COMMON HERBALS - EPICARDIUM

E	Energy - CoQ 10
P	Prostate – Saw Palmetto
I	Immune – Echinacea, Elderberry, Ginseng
C	Cholesterol – Fish Oil, Garlic, Niacin
A	Anxiety – Valerian root
R	Respiratory – Peppermint
D	Depression – St John's Wort
I	Insomnia – Melatonin
U	Urinary tract - Cranberry
M	Memory – Ginkgo, Menopause – Black cohosh

QUESTION S1.

Pregnant mothers generally need which supplement before conception to help prevent anencephaly and bifida?

a) Folic acid
b) Vitamin C
c) Vitamin D
d) Vitamin E

QUESTION S1.

Pregnant mothers generally need which supplement before conception to help prevent anencephaly and bifida?

a) **Folic acid**
b) Vitamin C
c) Vitamin D
d) Vitamin E

Answer: A. Folic acid. The American College of Obstetricians and Gynecologists recommend folic acid before conception and during early pregnancy to reduce neural tube defects risk.

If you were wondering, an obstetrician basically helps with everything up until immediately after delivery, while a gynecologist helps with women's health issues. An OB-GYN encompasses both.

QUESTION S2.

A patient looking for valerian root would most likely be trying to treat which condition?

    a) Anxiety
    b) High cholesterol
    c) Prostate issues
    d) Urinary tract issues

QUESTION S2.

A patient looking for valerian root would most likely be trying to treat which condition?

a) **Anxiety**
b) High cholesterol
c) Prostate issues
d) Urinary tract issues

Answer: A. Anxiety, the A in the epicardium mnemonic.

QUESTION S3.

A patient receives an oral contraceptive, which supplement would be of most concern?

 a) St. John's Wort
 b) Echinacea
 c) Vitamin C
 d) Vitamin D

QUESTION S3.

A patient receives an oral contraceptive, which supplement would be of most concern?

a) St. John's Wort
b) Echinacea
c) Vitamin C
d) Vitamin D

Answer: A. St. John's Wort. Because patients often don't consult a medical provider with OTCs and herbals, it's really important to ask the patient if they are on any vitamins or supplements, many think these are not medicines and don't count, but with interactions, they do.

QUESTION S4.

With Saw Palmetto, we expect the patient is trying to self-treat which condition?

a) BPH
b) CHF
c) ADHD
d) RA

QUESTION S4.

With Saw Palmetto, we expect the patient is trying to self-treat which condition?

a) **BPH**
b) CHF
c) ADHD
d) RA

Answer: A. BPH, benign prostatic hyperplasia. Whether in your mind's eye or on paper, write out abbreviations to have a more complete picture.

A. BPH, benign prostatic hyperplasia, a prostate gland enlargement.

B. CHF, congestive heart failure, where the heart either doesn't fill (diastolic pressure) or pump (systolic pressure) appropriately.

C. ADHD, Attention-deficit/hyperactivity disorder, is a concern with attention, hyperactivity and impulsive behaviors.

D. RA, Rhematoid arthritis, an inflammation of the joints caused by the immune system.

CHAPTER 9 PRACTICE DOSAGE CALCUATIONS QUESTIONS

QUESTION GD1.

A patient is to take bismuth subsalicylate liquid 2 tbsp PO q 1 hr for no greater than 8 doses in a day. What then, is the maximum daily dose in mL?

a) 60 mL
b) 120 mL
c) 240 mL
d) 300 mL

Question GD1.

A patient is to take bismuth subsalicylate liquid 2 tbsp PO q 1 hr for no greater than 8 doses in a day. What then, is the maximum daily dose in mL?

a) 60 mL/day
b) 120 mL/day
c) 240 mL/day
d) 300 mL/day

Answer: C, 240 mL/ day.

While I understand calculations are a real concern for most that take the exam, the most important thing to do is get a confident first step. Most calculations problems will have the units in the multiple-choice answer and except for alligations, can be solved by dimensional analysis, also known as the factor-label method. What we'll do in this book is standardize our process so you always know where to start your math solution.

Step 1: Draw your shoe bin. Your first step should be to draw a 4 by 2 table. It's actually easier to think of an 8-bin shoe organizer with four columns (up and down vertical) with two rows (side to side horizontal).

Microsoft Word: In Microsoft Word, you can click on "Table" then move to 4x2 and it will create this for you.

Paper and Pencil: If you are working with pencil and paper, you can make the fence where you create a horizontal line, then split that in half and those halves again which looks like a fence that has 4 columns and 2 rows. Either way, there are eight places to put numbers and units.

Step 2: Copy answer labels. Since this is a multiple-choice answer, we see that each answer has mL/day and we can put that in the furthest right column of our math shoe-bin organizer. This is such an important step because you have basically put the ending coordinates in your math GPS.

			mL
			day

Step 3: Write conversion factors. Remember, a conversion factor is a way to get from one factor to another. For example, 2.2 pounds / 1 kg is the same as 1 kg / 2.2 pounds. This is the hardest part of the problem because you have to change words into numbers. Once you get through here, you are in really good shape, but I'm going to show you why this can be hard. Our first factor in the problem is

|8 doses / 1 day |

That's easy to find, it says it right there in the problem. But what's a little harder to find is how many tablespoons there are in a single dose. It's not actually written in there, you have to understand that 2 tablespoons per hour is also 2 tablespoons per dose. That's our second conversion factor.

|2 tablespoons / 1 dose |

Our third conversion factor is one that, as a pharmacy technician, you are expected to memorize. There are 15 mL in 1 tablespoon.

|15 mL / 1 tablespoon |

Now let's put all our conversion factors together with our box and figure out where they belong.

|8 doses / 1 day | 2 tbsp / 1 dose |15 mL / 1 tbsp |

Step 4: Insert conversion factors

We start with 8 doses per 1 day because when we see our bin shoe organizer, day is on the bottom. We place the 8 doses per 1 day in the far left of our organizer. This process might feel a little like when you try pieces in a physical puzzle, some don't fit right and you have to try another.

8 doses			mL
1 day			1 day

But, now we see we have to somehow change doses to mL. We have a conversion factor for doses, that is, 1 dose / 2 tbsp. We can put that in next. We put dose on bottom because we want to cross it out, so it needs to be diagonal to the 8 doses.

8 ~~doses~~	2 tbsp		mL
1 day	1 ~~dose~~		1 day

We are closer, but need to now turn 2 tbsp into mL. We use our last conversion factor, 15 mL / 1 tbsp to do that crossing out the tbsp factor and leaving only mL and day.

8 ~~doses~~	2 ~~tbsp~~	15 **mL**	mL
1 **day**	1 ~~dose~~	1 ~~tbsp~~	1 day

Step 5: Complete the math. Now that we have all of our factors filled in, we can do the math and multiply 8 times 2 times 15 to get 240. Every number on the bottom is a 1, so if we divide by 1, we still get 240, our answer, 240 mL / day.

8 ~~doses~~	2 ~~tbsp~~	15 mL	240 mL
1 day	1 ~~dose~~	1 ~~tbsp~~	1 day

The most important thing in solving pharmacy technician math is to have the first steps, then to use what the problem gives you. If you look back on your math, it's probably a hot mess when you see it written out. However, by using the shoe-bin math organizer or fence method, I think it's a much better way to memorize the steps in the process.

Step 1: Draw your shoe bin.

Step 2: Copy answer labels.

Step 3: Write conversion factors.

Step 4: Insert conversion factors

Step 5: Complete the Math

At first, this process will feel slow, but as you get better at it, it will speed up and most importantly, improve your accuracy. We'll use this shoe-bin math as we continue throughout the book to practice.

QUESTION MD2.

A child needs 7.5 mL of ibuprofen over-the-counter liquid for pain every 6 hours around the clock. Each dose would then require how many tsp?

a) 1 tsp / dose
b) 1.5 tsp / dose
c) 2 tsp / dose
d) 2.5 tsp / dose

Question MD2.

A child needs 7.5 mL of ibuprofen over-the-counter liquid for pain every 6 hours around the clock. Each dose would then require how many tsp?

a) 1 tsp/dose
b) **1.5 tsp / dose**
c) 2 tsp /dose
d) 2.5 tsp /dose

Answer: B. 1.5 tsp.

Step 1: Draw your shoe bin.

Step 2: Copy answer labels.

			tsp
			dose

Step 3: Write conversion factors.

|7.5 mL / 1 dose | 1 tsp / 5 mL |

Step 4: Insert conversion factors

7.5 ~~mL~~	1 tsp		tsp
1 dose	5 ~~mL~~		dose

Step 5: Complete the Math

7.5 ~~mL~~	1 tsp		1.5 tsp
1 dose	5 ~~mL~~		dose

QUESTION RD3.

A patient pays cash for their prescription for albuterol with 200 metered puffs and wants to know how long it should last them. They say they've only been using 2 puffs three times a day on average instead of the four times a day the doctor said they might need. How long, in days, will this single inhaler last the patient using 2 puffs three times daily?

    a) 22
    b) 33
    c) 66
    d) 90

Question RD3.

A patient pays cash for their prescription for albuterol with 200 metered puffs and wants to know how long it should last them. They say they've only been using 2 puffs three times a day on average instead of the four times a day the doctor said they might need. How long, in days, will this single inhaler last the patient using 2 puffs three times daily?

    a) 22
    b) 33
    c) 66
    d) 90

Answer: B, 33 days.

Step 1: Draw your shoe bin.

Step 2: Copy answer labels.

			days
			inhaler

Step 3: Write conversion factors.

1 dose / 2 puffs | 1 day / 3 doses | 200 puffs / 1 inhaler |

Step 4: Insert conversion factors

200 puffs	1 dose	1 day	days
1 inhaler	2 puffs	3 doses	inhaler

Step 5: Complete the Math

200 ~~puffs~~	1 ~~dose~~	1 **day**	33 **days**
1 **inhaler**	2 ~~puffs~~	3 ~~doses~~	1 **inhaler**

QUESTION ID4.

A patient struggles to swallow pills and needs 500 mg of amoxicillin q 8 h for 14 days. How many Amoxicillin 250 mg/5 mL, 150 mL bottles will you dispense?

    a) 2
    b) 3
    c) 4
    d) 5

Question ID4.

A patient struggles to swallow pills and needs 500 mg of amoxicillin q 8 h for 14 days. How many Amoxicillin 250 mg/5 mL suspension in 150 mL bottles will you dispense?

  a) 2
  b) 3
  c) 4
  d) 5

Answer: C. 3.

Step 1: Draw your shoe bin.

Note, to solve this problem, you will need six columns.

Step 2: Copy answer labels.

14 days					bottles

Step 3: Write conversion factors.

| 3 doses / day | 500 mg / dose | 5 mL / 250 mg |

|1 bottle / 150 mg |

Step 4: Insert conversion factors

14 days	3 doses	500 mg	5 mL	1 bottle	bottles
	Day	Dose	250 mg	150 mL	

473

Step 5: Complete the Math

14 days	3 doses	500 mg	5 mL	1 bottle	2.8 bottles
	Day	Dose	250 mg	150 mL	

Now that I have that I need 2.8 bottles, I would have to round up a bit as there is no partial bottle when you are dispensing these kinds of prescriptions, so 3 bottles is the answer.

QUESTION ND5.

With phenytoin 125mg/5mL, the prescriber asks for 1 teaspoonful three times daily. How many mL would a patient need for 30 days' supply?

a) 120 mL
b) 300 mL
c) 450 mL
d) 600 mL

Question ND5.

With phenytoin 125mg/5mL, the prescriber asks for 1 teaspoonful three times daily. How many mL would a patient need for 30 days' supply?

a) 120 mL
b) 300 mL
c) **450 mL**
d) 600 mL

Answer: C. 450mL.

Step 1: Draw your shoe bin.

Step 2: Copy answer labels.

30 days			mL

Step 3: Write conversion factors.

| 5 mL / 1 teaspoonful | 3 teaspoonfuls / day |

Step 4: Insert conversion factors

30 days	3 tsp	5 mL	mL
	1 day	1 tsp	

Step 5: Complete the Math

30 days	3 tsp	5 mL	450 mL
	1 day	1 tsp	

QUESTION CD6.

A cardiac patient receives the following prescription. As the patient has high blood pressure, the prescriber will use a short course of treatment and taper the dosage as follows:

Methylprednisolone 4 mg tablets
Disp: 6 days' supply
Sig: 6 tabs PO day 1, 5 tabs PO day 2, 4 tabs PO day 3, 3 tabs PO day 4, 2 tabs PO day 5, and 1 tab po day 6.

How many tablets will the pharmacy need to dispense for this prescription?

a) 14
b) 21
c) 24
d) 42

Question CD6.

A cardiac patient receives the following prescription. As the patient has high blood pressure, the prescriber will use a short course of treatment and taper the dosage as follows:

Methylprednisolone 4 mg tablets
Disp: 6 days' supply
Sig: 6 tabs PO day 1, 5 tabs PO day 2, 4 tabs PO day 3, 3 tabs PO day 4, 2 tabs PO day 5, and 1 tab po day 6.

How many tablets will the pharmacy need to dispense for this prescription?

    a) 14
    b) 21
    c) 24
    d) 42

Answer: B. 21. This is one of those dreaded prescriptions to type out, but the math can actually be done with some quick addition that sounds a lot like a rocket ship countdown. I would take the extra minute to write out the addition so as not to make a preventable mistake.

$6 + 5 + 4 + 3 + 2 + 1 = 21$ tablets.

QUESTION ED7.

How many days will a Lantus SoloSTAR U-100 Pen last if there are 3 mL in the pen and the patient uses 20 units a day?

    a) 15
    b) 30
    c) 45
    d) 60

Question ED7.

How many days will a Lantus SoloSTAR U-100 Pen last if there are 3 mL in the pen and the patient uses 20 units a day?

    a) **15**
    b) 30
    c) 45
    d) 60

Answer: D. 15.

Step 1: Draw your shoe bin.

Step 2: Copy answer labels.

3 mL			days

Step 3: Write conversion factors.

100 Units / 1 mL which you have to memorize.

20 Units / day from the problem.

Step 4: Insert conversion factors

3 mL	100 units	1 day	days
	1 mL	20 units	

Step 5: Complete the Math

3 mL	100 units	1 day	15 days
	1 mL	20 units	

QUESTION D8.

A prescriber wants 2 mg per kg q.i.d. for a 220-pound patient. How many mg will the patient receive daily?

    a) 100
    b) 200
    c) 400
    d) 800

Question D8.

A prescriber wants 2 mg per kg q.i.d. for a 220-pound patient. How many mg will the patient receive daily?

 a) 100
 b) 200
 c) 400
 d) 800

Answer: D. 800.

Step 1: Draw your shoe bin with five columns.

Let's start by putting our shoe bin up with milligrams/day at the end and 220 pounds at the beginning so we have a clear picture of our starting and finishing line.

Step 2: Copy answer labels.

220 lbs.				mg
				day

Step 3: Write conversion factors.

Let's get our conversion factors. I use what are called pipes (it's on your keyboard above the slash) to separate them.

2.2 lbs. / 1 kg | 2 mg/kg/dose | 4 doses / day |

Now, some people like to figure out what the number of kilograms is in a separate equation, which is fine, but I'll show you how you can just make one single equation which makes it a lot easier to imagine in your mind's eye.

Step 4: Insert conversion factors

220 lbs.	1 kg	2 mg	4 doses	mg
	2.2 lbs.	kg / dose	day	day

Step 5: Complete the Math

220 lbs.	1 kg	2 mg	4 doses	800 mg
	2.2 lbs.	kg / dose	day	day

QUESTION D9.

A prescription arrives electronically at the pharmacy with the following instructions:

Sig: Two 250 mg tablets day one and then one tablet each day until all taken for four additional days

What is the dosage of the entire regimen?

    a) 500 mg
    b) 1000 mg
    c) 1200 mg
    d) 1500 mg

Question D9.

A prescription arrives electronically at the pharmacy with the following instructions:

Sig: Two 250 mg tablets day one and then one tablet each day until all taken for four additional days

What is the dosage of the entire regimen?

    a) 500 mg
    b) 1000 mg
    c) 1200 mg
    d) 1500 mg

Answer: D. 1500 mg.

You might recognize this as a Zithromax Z-Pak, but you'll be amazed at how many people put 5 tablets and then calculate milligrams incorrectly. Note, the first two tablets are a loading dose meant to get the drug levels above a certain range.

How many milligrams did the patient get in total? There's nothing wrong with adding $2 + 1 + 1 + 1 + 1 = 6$ to get the number of tablets they got in the regimen. You could do $((2*1) + (4*1)) = 6$, but that seems like you could make a mistake in that parenthesis madness. You do parenthesis first, multiplication, then addition. Once you know you need six tablets, set up the equation and solve.

6 tablets	250 mg	1500 mg
	1 tablet	

QUESTION D10.

How many milligrams will a patient be able to get from a 120 mL bottle of ibuprofen that has 100 mg/teaspoonful?

   a) 800
   b) 1600
   c) 2400
   d) 3200

Question D10.

How many milligrams will a patient be able to get from a 120 mL bottle of ibuprofen that has 100 mg/teaspoonful?

    a) 800
    b) 1600
    c) 2400
    d) 3200

Answer: C. 2400. You'll need to have a few measures memorized, but the math is straightforward.

Step 1: Draw your shoe bin with four columns.

Step 2: Copy answer labels.

120 mL			mg

Step 3: Write conversion factors.

| 5 mL / 1 tsp | 100 mg / 1 tsp |

Step 4: Insert conversion factors

120 mL	1 tsp	100 mg	mg
	5 mL	1 tsp	

Step 5: Complete the Math

120 mL	1 tsp	100 mg	2400 mg
	5 mL	1 tsp	

QUESTION D11.

A patient needs a month's supply of ibuprofen 800 milligrams that they take three times daily. How many tablets should be dispensed?

    a) 30
    b) 60
    c) 90
    d) 120

Question D11.

A patient needs a month's supply of ibuprofen 800 milligrams that they take three times daily. How many tablets should be dispensed?

    a) 30
    b) 60
    c) 90
    d) 120

Answer: C. 90.

Step 1: Draw your shoe bin with four columns.

Step 2: Copy answer labels.

1 month			tablets

Step 3: Write conversion factors.

| 3 tablets / 1 day |1 month / 30 days |

Step 4: Insert conversion factors

1 month	30 days	3 tablets	tablets
	1 month	1 day	

Step 5: Complete the Math

1 month	30 days	3 tablets	90 tablets
	1 month	1 day	

QUESTION D12.

What percentage of drug product do you get when you combine 60 g of 5% ointment with 15 g of 2% ointment?

a) 0.044 %
b) 0.44 %
c) 4.44 %
d) 44.4 %

Question D12.

What percentage of drug product do you get when you combine 60 g of 5% ointment with 15 g of 2% ointment?

    a) 0.044 %
    b) 0.44 %
    c) 4.44 %
    d) 44.4 %

Answer: C. 4.44%. There's actually a way to do this problem without doing any math at all. Many times, the test makers will try to trick you on decimals and put the exact same numbers in with the decimal moving in each case. However, the 2% and 5% represent the minimum and maximum of the ointment percentage.

For example, if you have 2% milk and 1% milk, there is no combination of those two milks that can take you below 1% or above 2%. It's mathematically impossible. Since the only number that falls between 2 and 5 is 4.44, that's the answer, but let me show you how to do the match anyway.

The first thing I would recommend is to not use decimals in the conversion. Instead of trying to get the 0.02 and 0.05 by dividing 2% and 5% by 100, then I would recommend using that a percent of anything is that number over 100.

60 g	5 g active	3 g	
	100 g cream		
15 g	2 g active	.3 g	
	100 g cream		
75 g total ointment		3.3 g active	

3.3 active / 75 g total = .044 x 100 = 4.4% in the new ointment mixture.

CHAPTER 10 MATCHING EXAMS

Congratulations! You've made it through the first 300 drugs in this book. I hope that you've started to commit the mnemonics to memory and found suffixes and prefixes you can count on to help you remember drug classes.

The following pages include two final pharmacology matching exams. The first final exam provides generic and brand names for the medications, and is a little easier. The second final exam, like some of your board exams, provides only generic names for a greater challenge.

If you feel you want more of a review, you can look at the summary of prefixes and suffixes in the index and then move on to the exams.

Remember to underline the drug stems first and picture what chapter you learned them in.

After you are done, review the ones you missed and shore up some memorization gaps.

MATCHING EXAM 1, QUESTIONS 1-25, CH. 1-3

___1 Loperamide (Imodium)
___2 Acetaminophen (Tylenol)
___3 Allopurinol (Zyloprim)
___4 APAP / Codeine (Tylenol/Codeine)
___5 Budesonide / Formoterol (Symbicort)
___6 Omeprazole (Prilosec)
___7 Esomeprazole (Nexium)
___8 Febuxostat (Uloric)
___9 Guaifenesin / Dextromethorphan (Robitussin DM)
__10 Fluticasone / Salmeterol (Advair)
__11 Hydrocodone / APAP (Vicodin)
__12 Fentanyl (Duragesic)
__13 Famotidine (Pepcid)
__14 Docusate sodium (Colace)
__15 Celecoxib (Celebrex)
__16 Aspirin [ASA] (Ecotrin)
__17 Alendronate (Fosamax)
__18 Albuterol (ProAir)
__19 ASA / APAP / Caffeine (Excedrin)
__20 Bismuth subsalicylate (Pepto-Bismol)
__21 Calcium carbonate (Tums)
__22 Guaifenesin / Codeine (Cheratussin AC)
__23 Cetirizine (Zyrtec)
__24 Diphenhydramine (Benadryl)
__25 Etanercept (Enbrel)

a. 1st-generation antihistamine	b. 2nd-generation antihistamine
c. 5-HT$_3$ receptor antagonist	d. Antacid
e. Anticholinergic for asthma	f. Anti-diarrheal
g. Anti-gout	h. Anti-nausea
i. Bisphosphonate	j. DMARD
k. H$_2$ blocker	l. Laxative
m. Expectorant/cough	n. Non-narcotic analgesic combo
o. Non-narcotic analgesic	p. NSAID
q. Opioid analgesic	r. Proton pump inhibitor
s. Short-acting bronchodilator	t. Steroid/bronchodilator

MATCHING EXAM 1, QUESTIONS 26-50, CH. 4

__26 Raltegravir (Isentress)
__27 Amoxicillin / Clavulanate (Augmentin)
__28 Ceftriaxone (Rocephin)
__29 Doxycycline (Doryx)
__30 Levofloxacin (Levaquin)
__31 Sulfamethoxazole / Trimethoprim (Bactrim)
__32 Cephalexin (Keflex)
__33 Ethambutol (Myambutol)
__34 Rifampin (Rifadin)
__35 Isoniazid (INH)
__36 Amikacin (Amikin)
__37 Cefepime (Maxipime)
__38 Amphotericin B (Fungizone)
__39 Amoxicillin (Amoxil)
__40 Azithromycin (Zithromax)
__41 Fluconazole (Diflucan)
__42 Oseltamivir (Tamiflu)
__43 Minocycline (Minocin)
__44 Clarithromycin (Biaxin)
__45 Gentamicin (Garamycin)
__46 Pyrazinamide (PZA)
__47 Nystatin (Mycostatin)
__48 Erythromycin (E-Mycin)
__49 Ciprofloxacin (Cipro)
__50 Acyclovir (Zovirax)

a. 1st-generation cephalosporin
b. 2nd-generation cephalosporin
c. 3rd-generation cephalosporin
d. 4th-generation cephalosporin
e. Antibiotic: aminoglycoside
f. Antibiotic: fluoroquinolone
g. Antibiotic: macrolide
h. Antibiotic: penicillin
i. Antibiotic: sulfa
j. Antibiotic: tetracycline
k. Antifungal
l. Antituberculosis
m. Antiviral: herpes
n. Antiviral: HIV
o. Antiviral: Influenza

__51 Sertraline (Zoloft)
__52 Carbamazepine (Tegretol)
__53 Cyclobenzaprine (Flexeril)
__54 Divalproex (Depakote)
__55 Gabapentin (Neurontin)
__56 Lithium (Lithobid)
__57 Meclizine (Antivert)
__58 Lidocaine (Solarcaine)
__59 Fluoxetine (Prozac)
__60 Escitalopram (Lexapro)
__61 Clonazepam (Klonopin)
__62 Benzocaine (Anbesol)
__63 Amitriptyline (Elavil)
__64 Atomoxetine (Strattera)
__65 Dexmethylphenidate (Focalin)
__66 Escitalopram (Lexapro)
__67 Haloperidol (Haldol)
__68 Lorazepam (Ativan)
__69 Levodopa / Carbidopa (Sinemet)
__70 Donepezil (Aricept)
__71 Citalopram (Celexa)
__72 Alprazolam (Xanax)
__73 Chlorpromazine (Thorazine)
__74 Eszopiclone (Lunesta)
__75 Isocarboxazid (Marplan)

a. ADHD drug/non-stimulant
b. ADHD drug/stimulant
c. Alzheimer's
d. Antidepressant: MAOI
e. Antidepressant: SNRI
f. Antidepressant: SSRI
g. Antidepressant: TCA
h. Antiepileptic: newer
i. Antiepileptic: traditional
j. Antipsychotic: 2nd generatio
k. Antipsychotic: 1st-generation
l. Benzodiazepine
m. Local anesthetic
n. Muscle relaxer
o. Parkinson's
p. Sedative-hypnotic
q. Simple salt
r. Vertigo/motion sickness

MATCHING EXAM 1, QUESTIONS 76-100, CH. 6-7

__76 Norethindrone / Ethinyl estradiol / Fe (Loestrin Fe)
__77 Bethanechol (Urecholine)
__78 Amlodipine (Norvasc)
__79 Diltiazem (Cardizem)
__80 Glucagon (GlucaGen)
__81 Finasteride (Proscar)
__82 Hydrochlorothiazide (Microzide)
__83 Regular insulin (Humulin R)
__84 HCTZ / Triamterene (Dyazide)
__85 Oxybutynin (Ditropan)
__86 Clopidogrel (Plavix)
__87 Norgestimate / Ethinyl estradiol (Tri-Sprintec)
__88 Propranolol (Inderal)
__89 Furosemide (Lasix)
__90 Enalapril (Vasotec)
__91 Insulin glargine (Lantus)
__92 Enoxaparin (Lovenox)
__93 Atorvastatin (Lipitor)
__94 Digoxin (Lanoxin)
__95 Norelgestromin / Ethinyl estradiol (OrthoEvra)
__96 Dutasteride (Avodart)
__97 Glipizide (Glucotrol)
__98 Heparin
__99 Glyburide (DiaBeta)
_100 Etonogestrel / Ethinyl estradiol (NuvaRing)

a. ACE inhibitor
b. ARB
c. Anticoagulant
d. Antidiabetic
e. Antiplatelet
f. Beta blocker
g. BPH: 5-alpha-reductase inhibitor
h. BPH: Alpha blocker
i. Calcium channel blocker
j. Cardiac glycoside
k. Contraception
l. Diuretic
m. For hypoglycemia
n. For hyperthyroidism
o. For hypothyroidism
p. HMG-CoA reductase inhib.
q. Erectile dysfunction
r. OAB
s. Longer duration insulin
t. Slower acting insulin
u. Urinary retention
v. Vasodilator

MATCHING EXAM 2, QUESTIONS 1-25, CH. 1-3

___1 Loratadine
___2 Diphenhydramine
___3 Nizatidine
___4 Pseudoephedrine
___5 Esomeprazole
___6 Naproxen
___7 Triamcinolone
___8 Infliximab
___9 Loperamide
__10 Bismuth subsalicylate
__11 Ibuprofen
__12 Magnesium hydroxide
__13 Methotrexate [MTX]
__14 Cetirizine
__15 Hydrocodone / APAP
__16 Prednisone
__17 Sumatriptan
__18 Tiotropium
__19 Promethazine
__20 Polyethylene glycol
__21 Oxycodone / APAP
__22 Omeprazole
__23 Ondansetron
__24 Morphine
__25 Methylprednisolone

a. 1st-generation antihistamine
b. 2nd-generation antihist.
c. 5-HT3 receptor antagonist
d. Antacid
e. Anticholinergic for asthma
f. Anti-diarrheal
g. Anti-gout
h. Anti-nausea
i. Decongestant
j. DMARD
k. H2 blocker
l. Laxative
m. Expectorant/cough
n. Non-narcotic analg. combo
o. Non-narcotic analgesic
p. NSAID
q. Opioid analgesic
r. Proton pump inhibitor
s. Steroid
t. Ulcerative colitis

MATCHING EXAM 2, QUESTIONS 26-50, CH. 4

__26 Doxycycline
__27 Amoxicillin
__28 SMZ / TMP
__29 Amphotericin B
__30 Erythromycin
__31 Ceftriaxone
__32 Rifampin
__33 Isoniazid
__34 Cephalexin
__35 Ethambutol
__36 Nystatin
__37 Minocycline
__38 Valacyclovir
__39 Zanamivir
__40 Amikacin
__41 Gentamicin
__42 Clarithromycin
__43 Cefepime
__44 Oseltamivir
__45 Fluconazole
__46 Ciprofloxacin
__47 Amoxicillin / Clavulanate
__48 Levofloxacin
__49 Pyrazinamide
__50 Darunavir

a. 1st-generation cephalosporin
b. 2nd-generation cephalospor.
c. 3rd-generation cephalosporin
d. 4th-generation cephalospor.
e. Antibiotic: aminoglycoside
f. Antibiotic: fluoroquinolone
g. Antibiotic: macrolide
h. Antibiotic: penicillin
i. Antibiotic: sulfa
j. Antibiotic: tetracycline
k. Antifungal
l. Antituberculosis
m. Antiviral: herpes
n. Antiviral: HIV
o. Antiviral: influenza

MATCHING EXAM 2, QUESTIONS 51-75, CH. 5

__51 Selegiline
__52 Sertraline
__53 Quetiapine
__54 Escitalopram
__55 Meclizine
__56 Isocarboxazid
__57 Gabapentin
__58 Levodopa / Carbidopa
__59 Memantine
__60 Phenytoin
__61 Ramelteon
__62 Citalopram
__63 Venlafaxine
__64 Trazodone
__65 Pregabalin
__66 Fluoxetine
__67 Lorazepam
__68 Haloperidol
__69 Lidocaine
__70 Paroxetine
__71 Risperidone
__72 Zolpidem
__73 Scopolamine
__74 Methylphenidate
__75 Lithium

a. ADHD drug / non-stimulant
b. ADHD drug/stimulant
c. Alzheimer's
d. Antidepressant: MAOI
e. Antidepressant: SNRI
f. Antidepressant: SSRI
g. Antidepressant: TCA
h. Antiepileptic: Newer
i. Antiepileptic: Traditional
j. Antipsychotic: 2nd-generat.
k. Antipsychotic: 1st-generation
l. Benzodiazepine
m. Local anesthetic
n. Muscle relaxer
o. Parkinson's
p. Sedative-hypnotic
q. Simple salt
r. Vertigo / motion sickness

MATCHING EXAM 2, QUESTIONS 76-100, CH. 6-7

__76 Levothyroxine
__77 Spironolactone
__78 Tolterodine
__79 Rosuvastatin
__80 Carvedilol
__81 Olmesartan
__82 Lovastatin
__83 Lisinopril
__84 Metformin
__85 Oxybutynin
__86 Atorvastatin
__87 Valsartan
__88 Tamsulosin
__89 Nifedipine
__90 Propylthiouracil
__91 Losartan
__92 Propranolol
__93 Tadalafil
__94 Sildenafil
__95 Verapamil
__96 Glipizide
__97 Enalapril
__98 Mannitol
__99 Metoprolol
__100. Warfarin

a. ACE inhibitor
b. Angiotensin receptor blocker
c. Anticoagulant
d. Antidiabetic
e. Antiplatelet
f. Beta blocker
g. BPH: 5-alpha-reductase inhib.
h. BPH: Alpha blocker
i. Calcium channel blocker
j. Cardiac glycoside
k. Contraception
l. Diuretic
m. For hypoglycemia
n. For hyperthyroidism
o. For hypothyroidism
p. HMG-CoA reductase inhibitor
q. Erectile dysfunction
r. OAB
s. Longer duration insulin
t. Slower acting insulin

CHAPTER 11 FULL DRUG LIST WITH SUFFIXES

CHAPTER 1 – GASTROINTESTINAL

I. Peptic Ulcer Disease

Antacids
Calcium Carbonate (Tums)
Magnesium Hydroxide (Milk of Magnesia)

Histamine-2 Receptor Antagonists (H$_2$RAs)
Cimetidine (Tagamet)
Famotidine (Pepcid, Zantac)
Nizatidine (Axid)

Proton Pump Inhibitors (PPIs)
Dexlansoprazole (Dexilant)
Esomeprazole (Nexium)
Omeprazole (Prilosec)
Lansoprazole (Prevacid)
Pantoprazole (Protonix)
Rabeprazole (AcipHex)

II. Diarrhea, IBS, constipation, and emesis

Antidiarrheals
Bismuth Subsalicylate (Pepto-Bismol)
Loperamide (Imodium)
Diphenoxylate / atropine (Lomotil)

Irritable bowel syndrome (IBS)
Dicyclomine (Bentyl)

Hyoscyamine (Anaspaz)

Constipation – Stool softener
Docusate sodium (Colace)

Constipation – Osmotic
Polyethylene glycol (PEG) 3350 (MiraLax)

Constipation – Miscellaneous
Lubiprostone (Amitiza)

Antiemetic – Serotonin 5-HT$_3$ receptor antagonist
Ondansetron (Zofran)

Antiemetic – Phenothiazine
Prochlorperazine (Compazine)
Promethazine (Phenergan)

III. Autoimmune disorders

Ulcerative colitis
Budesonide (Enterocort EC)
Infliximab (Remicade)

CHAPTER 2 – MUSCULOSKELETAL

I. NSAIDs and pain

OTC Analgesics – NSAIDs
Aspirin [ASA] (Ecotrin)
Ibuprofen (Advil, Motrin)
Naproxen (Aleve)

OTC Analgesic – Non-narcotic
Acetaminophen [APAP] (Tylenol)

OTC Migraine – NSAID / Non-narcotic analgesic
ASA/APAP/Caffeine (Excedrin Migraine)

RX Migraine – Narcotic and Non-narcotic analgesic
Butalbital / APAP / Caffeine (Fioricet)

RX Analgesics – NSAIDs
Diclofenac sodium extended release
    (Voltaren XR)
Etodolac (Lodine)
Indomethacin (Indocin)
Meloxicam (Mobic)
Nabumetone (Relafen)

RX Analgesics – NSAIDs – COX-2 inhibitor
Celecoxib (Celebrex)

II. Opioids and narcotics

Opioid analgesics – Schedule II
Morphine (Kadian, MS Contin)
Fentanyl (Duragesic, Sublimaze)
Hydrocodone / Acetaminophen (Vicodin)
Hydrocodone / Chlorpheniramine (Tussionex)

Hydrocodone / Ibuprofen (Vicoprofen)
Methadone (Dolophine)
Oxycodone (OxyIR, Oxycontin)
Oxycodone / Acetaminophen (Percocet)

Opioid analgesics - Schedule III
Acetaminophen w/codeine (Tylenol/codeine)

Mixed-opioid receptor analgesic – Schedule IV
Tramadol (Ultram)
Tramadol / Acetaminophen (Ultracet)

Opioid antagonist
Naloxone (Narcan)
Buprenorphine / Naloxone (Suboxone) [CIII]

III. Headaches and migraine

5-HT$_1$ receptor agonist
Eletriptan (Relpax)
Sumatriptan (Imitrex)

IV. DMARDs and rheumatoid arthritis

Methotrexate (Rheumatrex)
Abatacept (Orencia)
Etanercept (Enbrel)

V. Osteoporosis

Bisphosphonates
Alendronate (Fosamax)
Ibandronate (Boniva)
Risedronate (Actonel)

VI. Selective estrogen receptor modulator (SERM)

Raloxifene (Evista)

VII. Muscle relaxants

Baclofen (Lioresal)
Carisoprodol (Soma)
Cyclobenzaprine (Flexeril)
Diazepam (Valium)
Metaxalone (Skelaxin)
Methocarbamol (Robaxin)
Tizanidine (Zanaflex)

VIII. Gout

Colchicine (Colcrys)

Uric acid reducers
Allopurinol (Zyloprim)
Febuxostat (Uloric)

CHAPTER 3 – RESPIRATORY

I. Antihistamines and decongestants

Antihistamine – 1st-generation
Diphenhydramine (Benadryl)
Hydroxyzine (Atarax)

OTC Antihistamine – 2nd-generation
Cetirizine (Zyrtec)
Loratadine (Claritin)

OTC Antihistamine – 3nd generation
Fexofenadine (Allegra)
Levocetirizine (Xyzal)

OTC Antihistamine – Eye Drops
Olopatadine (Patanol, Pataday)

Antihistamine – Nasal Spray
Azelastine (Astelin)

OTC Antihistamine – 2nd generation /
Decongestant
Loratadine-D (Claritin-D)

BTC/OTC Decongestants
Pseudoephedrine (Sudafed) [BTC]
Phenylephrine (NeoSynephrine) [OTC]
Oxymetazoline (Afrin) [OTC]

II. Allergic rhinitis steroid, antitussives, and mucolytics

Allergic rhinitis steroid
Fluticasone (Flonase)
Mometasone nasal inhaler (Nasonex)

Triamcinolone (Nasacort Allergy 24HR)

OTC Antitussive / Mucolytic
Guaifenesin/DM (Mucinex DM, Robitussin DM)

RX Antitussive / Mucolytic
Guaifenesin / Codeine (Cheratussin AC)

RX Antitussive
Benzonatate (Tessalon Perles)

III. Asthma

Oral steroids
Dexamethasone (Decadron)
Methylprednisolone (Medrol)
Prednisone (Deltasone)

Ophthalmic steroid
Loteprednol ophthalmic (Lotemax)

Inhaled steroid / Beta$_2$ receptor agonist
Budesonide / Formoterol (Symbicort)
Fluticasone / Salmeterol (Advair)
Vilanterol / Umeclidinium (Anoro Ellipta)
Fluticasone / Vilanterol / Umeclidinium (Trelegy Ellipta)

Inhaled steroid
Budesonide (Rhinocort, Pulmicort Flexhaler)
Fluticasone (Flonase, Flovent HFA, Flovent Diskus)

Beta$_2$ receptor agonist short acting
Albuterol (ProAir HFA, Proventil)
Levalbuterol (Xopenex HFA)

Beta$_2$ receptor agonist / Anticholinergic

Albuterol / Ipratropium (DuoNeb)
Albuterol / Ipratropium (Combivent)

Anticholinergic
Tiotropium (Spiriva)

Leukotriene receptor antagonist
Montelukast (Singulair)

Anti-IgE antibody
Omalizumab (Xolair)

IV. Anaphylaxis

Epinephrine (EpiPen)

CHAPTER 4 – IMMUNE

I. OTC Antimicrobials

Antibiotic cream
Neomycin / Polymyxin B / Bacitracin (Neosporin)
Mupirocin (Bactroban) [RX]

Antifungal cream
Butenafine (Lotrimin Ultra)
Terbinafine (Lamisil)
Clotrimazole / Betamethasone (Lotrisone) [RX]

Vaccinations [Some RX, some antibacterial]
Influenza vaccine (Fluzone, Flumist)
Varicella (Varivax)
Zoster (Zostavax)

Antiviral OTC
Docosanol (Abreva)

II. Antibiotics that affect the cell wall

Penicillins
Amoxicillin (Amoxil)
Penicillin (Veetids)

Penicillin/Beta-lactamase inhibitor
Amoxicillin / Clavulanate (Augmentin)

Cephalosporins [by generation]
Cephalexin (Keflex) [1st]
Cefuroxime (Ceftin) [2nd]
Cefdinir (Omnicef) [3rd]
Ceftriaxone (Rocephin) [3rd]
Cefepime (Maxipime) [4th]

Ceftaroline (Teflaro) [5th]

Glycopeptide
Vancomycin (Vancocin)

III. Antibiotics – Protein Synthesis Inhibitors (Bacteriostatic)

Tetracyclines
Doxycycline (Doryx)
Minocycline (Minocin)
Tetracycline (Sumycin)

Macrolides
Azithromycin (Zithromax)
Clarithromycin (Biaxin)
Erythromycin (E-Mycin)
Fidaxomicin (Dificid)

Lincosamide
Clindamycin (Cleocin)

Oxazolidinone
Linezolid (Zyvox)

IV. Antibiotics – Protein Synth. Inhibitors (Bactericidal)

Aminoglycosides
Amikacin (Amikin)
Gentamicin (Garamycin)

V. Antibiotics for Urinary Tract Infections (UTIs) and Peptic Ulcer Disease (PUD)

OTC Urinary tract analgesic
Phenazopyridine (Uristat)

Nitrofuran
Nitrofurantoin (Macrobid, Macrodantin)

Dihydrofolate reductase inhibitor
Sulfamethoxazole / Trimethoprim (Bactrim DS)

Fluoroquinolones
Ciprofloxacin (Cipro)
Gatifloxacin ophthalmic (Zymar)
Levofloxacin (Levaquin)
Moxifloxacin (Avelox) / [Ophth. is Vigamox]

Nitroimidazole
Metronidazole (Flagyl)

VI. Anti-tuberculosis agents

Rifampin (Rifadin)
Isoniazid (INH)
Pyrazinamide (PZA)
Ethambutol (Myambutol)

VII. Antifungals

Amphotericin B (Fungizone)
Fluconazole (Diflucan)
Ketoconazole (Nizoral)
Nystatin (Mycostatin)

VIII. Antivirals – Non-HIV

Influenza A and B
Oseltamivir (Tamiflu)
Zanamivir (Relenza)

Herpes simplex virus & Varicella-Zoster Virus
HSV/VSV

Acyclovir (Zovirax)
Valacyclovir (Valtrex)

Respiratory Syncytial Virus RSV
156. Palivizumab (Synagis)

Hepatitis
Entecavir (Baraclude)
Hepatitis A (Havrix)
Hepatitis B (Recombivax HB)

HPV
Human papillomavirus (Gardasil)

IX. Antivirals – HIV

Fusion Inhibitor
Enfuvirtide (Fuzeon) (T-20)

CCR5 Antagonist
Maraviroc (Selzentry) (MVC)
Non-nucleoside reverse transcriptase inhibitors
(NNRTI) with two nucleoside / nucleotide reverse
transcriptase inhibitors (NRTIs)
Efavirenz (Sustiva) [NNRTI]
Emtricitabine / Tenofovir (Truvada) [NRTIs]
Efavirenz / Emtricitabine / Tenofovir (Atripla)
[NNRTI / NRTIs] (EFV / FTC / TDF)

Integrase Strand Transfer Inhibitor
Raltegravir (Isentress) (RAL)

Protease Inhibitor
Atazanavir (Reyataz) (ATV)
Darunavir (Prezista) (DRV)

X. Miscellaneous

Albendazole (Albenza) [Anthelmintic]
Hydroxychloroquine (Plaquenil) [Antimalarial]
Nitazoxanide (Alinia) [Antiprotozoal]

CHAPTER 5 – NEURO

I. OTC Local anesthetics and antivertigo

Local anesthetics
Benzocaine (Anbesol) [Ester type]
Lidocaine (Solarcaine) [Amide type]

Antivertigo
Meclizine (Dramamine, Antivert [RX])

II. Sedative-hypnotics (Sleeping pills)

OTC Non-narcotic analgesic / Sedative-hypnotic
Acetaminophen PM (Tylenol PM)

Benzodiazepine-like
Eszopiclone (Lunesta)
Zolpidem (Ambien)

Melatonin receptor agonist
Ramelteon (Rozerem)

Miscellaneous
Trazodone (Desyrel)

III. Antidepressants

Miscellaneous / SSRI
Vilazodone (Viibryd)

Selective serotonin reuptake inhibitors (SSRIs)
Citalopram (Celexa)
Escitalopram (Lexapro)
Sertraline (Zoloft)
Fluoxetine (Prozac, Sarafem)

Paroxetine (Paxil, Paxil CR)

Serotonin-Norepinephrine reuptake inhibitors (SNRIs)
Duloxetine (Cymbalta)
Desvenlafaxine (Pristiq)
Venlafaxine (Effexor)

Tricyclic antidepressants (TCAs)
Amitriptyline (Elavil)
Doxepin (Sinequan)
Nortriptyline (Pamelor)

Tetracycylic antidepressant (TeCA) Noradrenergic and specific serotonergic antidepressants (NaSSAs)
Mirtazapine (Remeron)

Monoamine oxidase inhibitor (MAOI)
Isocarboxazid (Marplan)

IV. Smoking Cessation

Bupropion (Wellbutrin, Zyban)
Varenicline (Chantix)

V. Barbiturates

196. Phenobarbital (Luminal)

VI. Benzodiazepines

Clonazepam (Klonopin)
Alprazolam (Xanax)
Lorazepam (Ativan)
Midazolam (Versed)
Temazepam (Restoril)

VII. Non-benzodiazepine / non-barbiturate

Bu<u>spir</u>one (Buspar)

VIII. ADHD medications

<u>Stimulant – Schedule II</u>
Am<u>phet</u>amine/Dextroam<u>phet</u>amine (Adderall)
Dexmethylphenidate (Focalin)
Lisdexam<u>fetamine</u> (Vyvanse)
Methylphenidate (Concerta)

<u>Non-stimulant – non-scheduled</u>
Atom<u>oxetine</u> (Strattera)

IX. Bipolar Disorder

<u>Simple salt</u>
Lithium (Lithobid)

XI. Schizophrenia

<u>First generation antipsychotic (FGA) (low potency)</u>
Chlorpromazine (Thorazine)

<u>First generation antipsychotic (FGA) (high potency)</u>
Halo<u>per</u>idol (Haldol)

<u>Second-generation antipsychotic (SGA)</u>
Ari<u>pipr</u>azole (Abilify)
Clozapine (Clozaril)
Olanza<u>pine</u> (Zyprexa)
Ris<u>per</u>idone (Risperdal)
Que<u>tia</u>pine (Seroquel)
Zipra<u>sidone</u> (Geodon)

XII. Antiepileptics

Traditional antiepileptics
Carbamazepine (Tegretol)
Divalproex (Depakote)
Phenytoin (Dilantin)

Newer antiepileptics
Gabapentin (Neurontin)
Lamotrigine (Lamictal)
Levetiracetam (Keppra)
Oxcarbazepine (Trileptal)
Pregabalin (Lyrica)
Topiramate (Topamax)

XIII. Parkinson's, Alzheimer's, Motion sickness

Parkinson's
Benztropine mesylate (Cogentin)
Levodopa / Carbidopa (Sinemet)
Selegiline (Eldepryl)
Pramipexole (Mirapex ER)
Ropinirole (Requip, Requip XL)

Alzheimer's
Donepezil (Aricept)
Memantine (Namenda)

Motion sickness
Scopolamine (Transderm-Scop)

CHAPTER 6 – CARDIO

I. OTC Antihyperlipidemics and antiplatelet

Antihyperlipidemics
Omega-3-acid ethyl esters (Lovaza)

Niacin (Niaspan ER)

<u>Antiplatelet</u>
Aspirin (Ecotrin)

II. Diuretics

<u>Osmotic</u>
Mannitol (Osmitrol)

<u>Loop</u>
Furosemide (Lasix)

<u>Thiazide</u>
Hydrochlorothiazide (Microzide)

<u>Potassium sparing and thiazide</u>
Triamterene/Hydrochlorothiazide (Dyazide)

<u>Potassium sparing</u>
Spironolactone (Aldactone)

<u>Electrolyte replenishment</u>
Potassium chloride (K-DUR)

III. Understanding the Alphas and Betas

<u>Alpha-1 antagonist</u>
Doxazosin (Cardura)
Terazosin (Hytrin)

<u>Alpha-2 agonist</u>
Clonidine (Catapres)

<u>Beta-blocker – 1st-generation – non-beta selective</u>
Propranolol (Inderal)

<u>Beta-blockers – 2nd-generation – beta selective</u>
Ate<u>nolol</u> (Tenormin)
Ate<u>nolol</u> / Chlorthalidone (Tenoretic)
Bisop<u>rolol</u> / Hydroch<u>lorothiazide</u> (Ziac)
Metop<u>rolol</u> succinate (Toprol-XL)
Metop<u>rolol</u> tartrate (Lopressor)

<u>Beta-blocker – 3rd-generation – non-beta selective</u>
<u>vasodilating</u>
Carve<u>dilol</u> (Coreg)
Labet<u>alol</u> (Normodyne)
Nebiv<u>olol</u> (Bystolic)

IV. Renin-angiotensin-aldosterone system (RAAS)

<u>ACE Inhibitors (ACEIs)</u>
Benaze<u>pril</u> / HCTZ (Lotensin HCT)
Enala<u>pril</u> (Vasotec)
Fosino<u>pril</u> (Monopril)
Quina<u>pril</u> (Accupril)
Lisino<u>pril</u> (Zestril)
Lisino<u>pril</u> / Hydroch<u>lorothiazide</u> (Zestoretic)
Rami<u>pril</u> (Altace)

<u>Angiotensin II receptor blockers (ARBs)</u>
Cande<u>sartan</u> (Atacand)
Irbe<u>sartan</u> (Avapro)
Irbe<u>sartan</u> / Hydroch<u>lorothiazide</u> (Avalide)
Lo<u>sartan</u> (Cozaar)
Lo<u>sartan</u> / Hydroch<u>lorothiazide</u> (Hyzaar)
Olme<u>sartan</u> (Benicar)
Olme<u>sartan</u> / HCTZ (Benicar HCT)
Telmi<u>sartan</u> / HCTZ (Micardis HCT)
Val<u>sartan</u> (Diovan)
Val<u>sartan</u> / HCTZ (Diovan HCT)

Angiotensin Receptor Neprilysin Inhibitor (ARNI)
Valsartan / Sacubitril (Entresto)

V. Calcium channel blockers (CCBs)

Non-dihydropyridines
Diltiazem (Cardizem)
Verapamil (Calan)

Dihydropyridines
Amlodipine (Norvasc)
Amlodipine / Atorvastatin (Caduet)
Amlodipine / Benazepril (Lotrel)
Amlodipine / Valsartan (Exforge)
Felodipine (Plendil)
Nifedipine (Procardia)

VI. Vasodilators

Hydralazine (Apresoline)
Isosorbide mononitrate (Imdur)
Nitroglycerin (Nitrostat)

VII. Anti-anginal

Ranolazine (Ranexa)

VIII. Antihyperlipidemics

HMG-CoA reductase inhibitors
Atorvastatin (Lipitor)
Lovastatin (Mevacor)
Pravastatin (Pravachol)
Rosuvastatin (Crestor)
Simvastatin (Zocor)

Fibric acid derivatives

Fenofibrate (Tricor)
Gemfibrozil (Lopid)

Bile acid sequestrant
Colesevelam (Welchol)

Cholesterol absorption blocker
Ezetimibe (Zetia)
Ezetimibe / Simvastatin (Vytorin)

IX. Anticoagulants and antiplatelets

Anticoagulants
Enoxaparin (Lovenox)
Heparin
Warfarin (Coumadin)
Dabigatran (Pradaxa)
Rivaroxaban (Xarelto)
Apixaban (Eliquis)

Antiplatelet
Aspirin / Dipyridamole (Aggrenox)
Clopidogrel (Plavix)
Prasugrel (Effient)
Ticagrelor (Brilinta)

X. Cardiac glycoside and Anticholinergic

Cardiac glycoside
Digoxin (Lanoxin)

Anticholinergic
Atropine (AtroPen)

XI. Antidysrhythmic
Amiodarone (Cordarone)

Memorizing Pharmacology

Chapter 7 – Endocrine / Misc.

I. OTC Insulin and emergency contraception

306. Regular Insulin (Humulin R)
307. NPH Insulin (Humulin N)
308. Levonorgestrel (Plan B One-Step)

II. Diabetes and insulin

Biguanides
Metformin (Glucophage)
Metformin / Glyburide (Glucovance)

DPP-4 Inhibitors (Gliptins)
Linagliptin (Tradjenta)
Saxagliptin (Onglyza)
Sitagliptin (Januvia)

Meglitinides (Glinides)
Repaglinide (Prandin)

Sulfonylureas – 2nd-generation
Glyburide (DiaBeta)
Glimepiride (Amaryl)
Glipizide (Glucotrol)

Thiazolidinediones (Glitazones)
Pioglitazone (Actos)
Rosiglitazone (Avandia)

Incretin mimetics
Exenatide (Byetta)
Liraglutide (Victoza)

Hypoglycemia

Glucagon (GlucaGen)

<u>RX Insulin</u>
Insulin aspart (Novolog)
Insulin lispro (Humalog)
Insulin detemir (Levemir)
Insulin glargine (Lantus, Toujeo)

III. Thyroid hormones

<u>Hypothyroidism</u>
Levothyroxine (Synthroid)

<u>Hyperthyroidism</u>
Propylthiouracil (PTU)

IV. Hormones and contraception

<u>Low testosterone</u>
Testosterone (AndroGel)

<u>Estrogens and / or Progestins</u>
Estradiol (Estrace, Estraderm)
Conjugated estrogens (Premarin)
Conjugated estrogens / Medroxyprogesterone
        (Prempro, Premphase)
Progesterone (Prometrium)
Medroxyprogesterone (Provera)

<u>Combined oral contraceptive pill (COCP)</u>
Ethinyl estradiol / norethindrone / Fe
(Loestrin 24 Fe)
Ethinyl estradiol / norgestimate (Tri-Sprintec)

<u>Patch</u>
Ethinyl estradiol / norelgestromin (OrthoEvra)

Ring
Ethinyl estradiol / etonogestrel (NuvaRing)

V. Overactive bladder, urinary retention, erectile dysfunction (ED), benign prostatic hyperplasia (BPH)

Overactive bladder
Oxybutynin (Ditropan)
Darifenacin (Enablex)
Solifenacin (VESIcare)
Tolterodine (Detrol)

Urinary retention
Bethanechol (Urecholine)

Erectile dysfunction - PDE-5 inhibitors
Sildenafil (Viagra)
Vardenafil (Levitra)
Tadalafil (Cialis)

BPH – Alpha-blocker
Alfuzosin (Uroxatral)
Tamsulosin (Flomax)

BPH – 5-alpha-reducase inhibitor
Dutasteride (Avodart)
Finasteride (Proscar, Propecia)

CHAPTER 12 THE OTC SCAVENGER HUNT

I learned drug names by working in a pharmacy. I recommend you start learning them with this lab activity. Medications you have held will be easier to memorize. If you are in the car driving and listening to the audio version of this book, obviously, just keep going, but I encourage you to try this activity when you have a chance.

Picture finding the drugs in an alphabetical list. It's not very conducive to memorization.

Acetaminophen	Famotidine	Neomycin /
Acetaminophen PM	Guaifenesin/DM	Polymyxin B /
ASA/APAP/Caffeine	Ibuprofen	Bacitracin
Aspirin (Low Dose)	Influenza vaccine	Niacin
Aspirin (Regular)	NPH insulin	Omega-3 E.E.
Benzocaine	Regular insulin	Omeprazole
Bismuth subsalicylate	Levonorgestrel	Oxymetazoline
Butenafine	Lidocaine	Phenylephrine
Calcium carbonate	Loperamide	Polyethylene gly.
Cetirizine	Loratadine	Pseudoephedrine
Diphenhydramine	Loratadine-D	Nizatidine
Docosanol	Magnesium hydroxide	Triamcinolone
Docusate sodium	Meclizine	
Esomeprazole	Naproxen	

Now picture (or actually find) this list sorted by pathophysiologic class. This is how pharmacies sort over-the-counter (OTC) drugs for placement on drug store shelves.

Gastrointestinal

Calcium carbonate	Esomeprazole	Docusate sodium
Magnesium hydroxide	Omeprazole	Polyethylene gly.

| Famotidine | Bismuth subsalicylate |
| Nizatidine | Loperamide |

Musculoskeletal
Aspirin (Regular)	Acetaminophen
Ibuprofen	Acetaminophen / Aspirin / Caffeine
Naproxen	

Respiratory
Diphenhydramine	Loratadine-D	Oxymetazoline
Cetirizine	Pseudoephedrine	Triamcinolone
Loratadine	Phenylephrine	Guaifenesin / DM

Immune
Neomycin /	Butenafine
Polymyxin B /	Docosanol
Bacitracin	Influenza vaccine

Neuro
| Benzocaine | Meclizine | Acetaminophen PM |
| Lidocaine | | |

Cardio
| Omega-3-Fatty E.E. | Niacin | Aspirin (Low Dose) |

Endocrine
| Regular insulin | NPH insulin | Levonorgestrel |

You will find the second list often grouped together in the pharmacy aisles. The same is true in your brain. It remembers drugs in related groups, not in strict alphabetical order, a better way to remember them.

APPENDIX

ANSWERS TO DRUG QUIZZES (LEVEL 1)

Gastrointestinal drugs
1. A 2. E 3. D 4. E 5. F 6. B 7. A/D 8. G 9. F 10. C
2. –tidine 4. –tidine 5. –prazole 8. –liximab 9. –prazole
10. -setron

Musculoskeletal drugs
1. E 2. C 3. F 4. B 5. D 6. I 7. I 8. G 9. H 10. A
2. –dronate 4. –xostat 5. –nercept 8. –profen 9. –coxib
10. -triptan

Respiratory drugs
1. I 2. B 3. A 4. J 5. F 6. C 7. B 8. E 9. D 10. G
1. –terol 4. –terol 6. –tropium 7. –atadine 8. –lukast
9. –drine 10. -pred-

Immune system drugs
1. H 2. G 3. D 4. C 5. K 6. E 7. L 8. F 9. K 10. M
1. –cillin 2. –thromycin 3. Cef- 4. Cef- 5. –conazole
6. –micin 8. -floxacin 10. –cyclovir

Nervous system drugs
1. K 2. F 3. A 4. E 5. B 6. H 7. J 8. C 9. L 10. M
1. –azolam 2. -triptyline 3. –oxetine 7. –peridol 9. –dopa
10. –pidem

Cardio system drugs
1. O 2. E 3. A 4. D 5. K 6. N 7. C 8. F 9. H 10. M
1. –vastatin 2. –grel 3. –pril 4. –parin 5. –semide
6. -thiazide 7. –sartan 8. –olol 9. –dipine

Endocrine / Misc. system drugs
1. A 2. H 3. A 4. M 5. I 6. A 7. J 8. N 9. L 10. K
1. Gli- 3. Gly- 6. –formin 9. –fenacin 10. –afil

ANSWERS TO DRUG QUIZZES (LEVEL 2)

Gastrointestinal drugs
1. B 2. F 3. F 4. D 5. C 6. A 7. E 8. D 9. B 10. E
1. -sal- 2. –prazole 3. –prazole 7. –tidine 10. –tidine

Musculoskeletal drugs
1. D 2. I 3. D 4. G 5. B 6. C 7. B 8. G 9. C 10. I
1. –trexate 3. –tacept 5. –xostat 6. -dronate 9. -dronate

Respiratory drugs
1. J 2. F 3. H 4. J 5. D 6. B 7. A 8. I 9. E 10. G
1. –terol 4. –terol 5. –drine 8. –terol 9. –lukast 10. Pred-

Immune system drugs
1. L 2. K 3. E 4. F 5. L 6. M 7. A 8. I 9. G 10. O
1. Rif- 3. –kacin 4. –floxacin 6. –cyclovir 7. Ceph-
8. Sulfa- / -prim 9. –thromycin 10. -amivir

Nervous system drugs
1. D 2. K 3. H 4. I 5. C 6. M 7. E 8. E 9. L 10. N
1. –faxine 2. –azepam 3. –toin 4. –tiapine 6. –clone
7. –oxetine 9. –giline

Cardio system drugs
1. I 2. G 3. C 4. N 5. B 6. H 7. P 8. A 9. J 10. D
1. –tiazem 2. –dil- (-olol) 3. –sartan 4. –thiazide 5. –azosin
6. –dipine 7. Nitro- 8. –pril 10. –farin

Endocrine / Misc. system drugs
1. B 2. C 3. L 4. K 5. E 6. F 7. L 8. O 9. K 10. B
1. –steride 4. –afil 5. estr- 6. -gest- / estr 9. –afil 10. -steride

ANSWERS TO FINAL EXAM (LEVEL 1)

1	f	26	n	51	f	76	k
2	o	27	h	52	i	77	u
3	g	28	c	53	n	78	i
4	q	29	j	54	i	79	i
5	t	30	f	55	h	80	m
6	r	31	i	56	q	81	g
7	r	32	a	57	r	82	l
8	g	33	l	58	m	83	t
9	m	34	l	59	f	84	l
10	t	35	l	60	f	85	r
11	q	36	e	61	l	86	e
12	q	37	d	62	m	87	k
13	k	38	k	63	g	88	f
14	l	39	h	64	a	89	l
15	p	40	g	65	b	90	a
16	p	41	k	66	f	91	s
17	i	42	o	67	k	92	c
18	s	43	j	68	l	93	p
19	n	44	g	69	o	94	j
20	f	45	e	70	c	95	k
21	d	46	l	71	f	96	g
22	m	47	k	72	l	97	d
23	b	48	g	73	k	98	c
24	a	49	f	74	p	99	d
25	j	50	m	75	d	100	k

ANSWERS TO FINAL EXAM (LEVEL 2)

1	b	26	j	51	o	76	o
2	a	27	h	52	f	77	l
3	k	28	i	53	j	78	r
4	i	29	k	54	f	79	p
5	r	30	g	55	r	80	f
6	p	31	c	56	d	81	b
7	s	32	l	57	h	82	p
8	t	33	l	58	o	83	a
9	f	34	a	59	c	84	d
10	f	35	l	60	i	85	r
11	p	36	k	61	p	86	p
12	d	37	j	62	f	87	b
13	j	38	m	63	e	88	h
14	b	39	o	64	p	89	i
15	q	40	e	65	h	90	n
16	s	41	e	66	f	91	b
17	c	42	g	67	l	92	f
18	e	43	d	68	k	93	q
19	h	44	o	69	m	94	q
20	l	45	k	70	f	95	i
21	q	46	f	71	j	96	d
22	r	47	h	72	p	97	a
23	h	48	f	73	r	98	l
24	q	49	l	74	b	99	f
25	s	50	n	75	q	100	c

ALPHABETICAL LIST OF STEMS

ac	anti-inflammatory agents (<u>ac</u>etic <u>ac</u>id derivatives)
adol	analgesics (mixed opiate receptor agonists/antagonists)
afil	phosphodiesterase type 5 (PDE5) inhibitors
alol	combined alpha and beta blockers
amivir	neuraminidase inhibitors
astine	antihistaminics (histamine-H$_1$ receptor antagonists)
atadine	tricyclic histaminic-H$_1$ receptor antagonists, lor<u>ata-dine</u> derivatives (formerly -tadine)
azepam	antianxiety agents (di<u>azepam</u> type)
azolam	(WHO stem) diazepam derivatives
azosin	antihypertensives (pr<u>azosin</u> type)
barb	<u>barb</u>ituric acid derivatives
bendazole	anthelmintics (ti<u>bendazole</u> type)
caine	local anesthetics
cavir	carbocyclic nucleosides
cef	cephalosporins
citabine	nucleoside antiviral / antineoplastic agents, cytarabine or azarabine derivatives
cillin	peni<u>cillin</u>s
clone	hypnotics/tranquilizers (zopi<u>clone</u> type)
conazole	systemic antifungals (mi<u>conazole</u> type)
coxib	cyclooxygenase-2 inhibitors
cycline	antibiotics (tetra<u>cycline</u> derivatives)
cyclovir	antivirals (a<u>cyclovir</u> type)
dil	vaso<u>dil</u>ators (undefined group)
dipine	phenylpyridine vasodilators (nife<u>dipine</u> type)
dopa	<u>dopa</u>mine receptor agonists
dralazine	antihypertensives (hy<u>dralazine</u>-phthalazines)
drine	sympathomimetics

APPENDIX

dronate	calcium metabolism regulators
estr	<u>estr</u>ogens
farin	war<u>farin</u> analogs
faxine	antianxiety, antidepressant inhibitor of norepinephrine and dopamine re-uptake
fenacin	muscarinic receptor antagonists
fetamine	am<u>fetamine</u> derivatives
fibrate	antihyperlipidemics (clo<u>fibrate</u> type)
floxacin	fluoroquinolone (not on Stem List)
formin	hypoglycemics (phen<u>formin</u> type)
gab	<u>gab</u>amimetics
gatran	thrombin inhibitors (ar<u>gatran</u> type)
gest	pro<u>gest</u>ins
giline	Monoamine oxidase (MAO) inhibitors, type B
gli (was gly)	antihyperglycemics
glinide	antidiabetic, sodium glucose co-transporter 2 (SGLT2) inhibitors, not phlorozin derivatives
gliptin	dipeptidyl aminopeptidase-IV inhibitors
glitazone	peroxisome proliferator activating receptor (PPAR) agonists (thiazolidene derivatives)
glutide	<u>glu</u>cagon-like pep<u>tide</u> (GLP) analogs
gly	antihyper<u>gly</u>cemics
grel	platelet aggregation inhibitors, primarily platelet P2Y12 receptor antagonists
icam	anti-inflammatory agents (isoxi<u>cam</u> type)
ifene	antiestrogens of the clom<u>ifene</u> and tamox<u>ifen</u> groups
imibe	antihyperlipidaemics, acyl CoA: cholesterol acyltransferase (ACAT) inhibitors
iodarone	indicates high iodine content antiarrhythmic
kacin	antibiotics obtained from *Streptomyces kanamyceticus* (related to <u>kanamy</u>cin)

liximab	monoclonal antibodies
lizumab	monoclonal antibodies
lukast	leukotriene receptor antagonists
mantine	antivirals/antiparkinsonians (adamantane derivatives)
melteon	selective melatonin receptor agonist
methacin	anti-inflammatory agents (indo<u>methacin</u> type)
micin	antibiotics (*Micromonospora* strains)
mycin	antibiotics (*Streptomyces* strain)
nal	narcotic agonists/antagonists (normorphine type)
navir	HIV protease inhibitors (saqui<u>navir</u> type)
nercept	tumor necrosis factor receptors
nicline	<u>ni</u>cotinic acetylcho<u>line</u> receptor partial agonists/agonists
nidazole	antiprotozoal substances (metro<u>nidazole</u> type)
nifur	5-<u>nitrofur</u>an derivatives
nitro	(WHO stem) NO_2 derivatives
olol	beta-blockers (propran<u>olol</u> type)
orphan	narcotic antagonists/agonists (m<u>orphinan</u> derivatives)
oxacin	antibacterials (quinolone derivatives)
oxanide	antiparasitics (salicylanilide derivatives)
oxetine	antidepressants (flu<u>oxetine</u> type)
pamil	coronary vasodilators (vera<u>pamil</u> type)
parin	he<u>parin</u> derivatives and low molecular weight (or depolymerized) heparins
peg	<u>PEG</u>ylated compounds, covalent attachment of macrogol (pol<u>ye</u>thylene <u>g</u>lycol) polymer
peridol	antipsychotics (halo<u>peridol</u> type)
peridone	antipsychotics (ris<u>peridone</u> type)
pezil	acetylcholinesterase inhibitors used in the treatment of Alzheimer's disease

APPENDIX

pidem	hypnotics/sedatives (zol<u>pidem</u> type)
pin(e)	tricyclic compounds
piprazole	(WHO stem) psychotropics, phenylpiperazine derivatives (future use is discouraged due to conflict with stem -prazole)
prazole	antiulcer agents (benzimidazole derivatives)
pred	<u>pred</u>nisone and <u>pred</u>nisolone derivatives
pril	antihypertensives (ACE inhibitors)
prim	antibacterials (trimetho<u>prim</u> type)
profen	anti-inflammatory/analgesic agents (ibu<u>profen</u> type)
prost	<u>prost</u>aglandins
racetam	nootropic agents (learning, cognitive enhancers), pi<u>racetam</u> type
rifa	antibiotics (<u>rifa</u>mycin derivatives)
sal	anti-inflammatory agents (<u>sal</u>icylic acid derivatives)
sartan	angiotensin II receptor antagonists
semide	diuretics (furo<u>semide</u> type)
setron	serotonin 5-HT$_3$ receptor antagonists
sidone	antipsychotic with binding activity on serotonin (5-HT2A) and dopamine (D2) receptors
spirone	anxiolytics (bu<u>spirone</u> type)
ster	<u>ster</u>oids (androgens, anabolics)
steride	testosterone reductase inhibitors
sulfa	antimicrobials (<u>sulfa</u>mides derivatives)
tacept	<u>T</u>-cell re<u>cept</u>ors
tegravir	int<u>egra</u>se inhibitors
terol	bronchodilators (phenethylamine derivatives)
thiazide	diuretics (<u>thiazide</u> derivatives)
thromycin	macrolide (not on Stem List)
tiapine	antipsychotics (dibenzo<u>thiaze</u><u>pine</u> derivatives)
tiazem	calcium channel blockers (dil<u>tiazem</u> type)

tide	pep<u>tide</u>s
tidine	H$_2$-receptor antagonists (cime<u>tidine</u> type)
toin	antiepileptics (hydan<u>toin</u> derivatives)
traline	selective serotonin reuptake inhibitors (SSRI)
trexate	antimetabolites (folic acid derivatives)
tril	endopeptidase inhibitors (e.g. neprilysin)
triptan	antimigraine agents (5-HT$_1$ receptor agonists); suma<u>triptan</u> derivatives
triptyline	antidepressants (dibenzol[a.d.]cycloheptane derivatives)
trop(ium)	<u>atrop</u>ine derivative, (quaternary ammonium salt)
trop(ine)	<u>atrop</u>ine derivatives; Subgroups: tertiary amines (e.g., benztropine)
uracil	<u>uracil</u> derivatives used as thyroid antagonists and as antineoplastics
vastatin	antihyperlipidemics (HMG-CoA inhibitors)
vir	anti<u>vir</u>als
virenz	non-nucleoside reverse transcriptase inhibitors; benzoxazinone derivatives
viroc	CC chemokine receptor type 5 (CCR5) antagonists
vudine	antineoplastics; antivirals (zido<u>vudine</u> group) (exception: edoxudine)
xaban	antithrombotics, blood coagulation factor XA inhibitors
xostat	xanthine oxidase/dehydrogenase inhibitors
zolid	oxa<u>zolid</u>inone antibacterials

LIST OF STEMS BY PHYSIOLOGIC CLASS

Chapter 1: Gastrointestinal

liximab	monoclonal antibodies
peg	PEGylated compounds, covalent attachment of macrogol (poly<u>e</u>thylene <u>g</u>lycol) polymer
prazole	antiulcer agents (benzimid<u>azole</u> derivatives)
prost	<u>prost</u>aglandins
sal	anti-inflammatory agents (<u>sal</u>icylic acid derivatives)
setron	serotonin 5-HT$_3$ receptor antagonists
tidine	H$_2$-receptor antagonists (cime<u>tidine</u> type)

Chapter 2: Musculoskeletal

ac	anti-inflammatory agents (<u>ac</u>etic <u>ac</u>id derivatives)
adol	analgesics (mixed opiate receptor agonists/antagonists)
coxib	cycl<u>oox</u>ygenase-2 inhibitors
dronate	calcium metabolism regulators
icam	anti-inflammatory agents (isox<u>icam</u> type)
ifene	antiestrogens of the clom<u>ifene</u> and tamox<u>ifen</u> groups
liximab	monoclonal antibodies
methacin	anti-inflammatory agents (indo<u>methacin</u> type)
nal	narcotic agonists/antagonists (normorphine type)
nercept	tumor necrosis factor receptors
profen	anti-inflammatory/analgesic agents (ibu<u>profen</u> type)
tacept	<u>T</u>-cell re<u>cept</u>ors
trexate	antimetabolites (folic acid derivatives)
triptan	antimigraine agents (5-HT$_1$ receptor agonists); suma<u>triptan</u> derivatives
xostat	xanthine oxidase/dehydrogenase inhibitors

Chapter 3: Respiratory

atadine	tricyclic histaminic-H₁ receptor antagonists, lo<u>ratadine</u> derivatives (formerly -tadine)
astine	antihistaminics (histamine-H₁ receptor antagonists)
drine	sympathomimetics
lizumab	monoclonal antibodies
lukast	leukotriene receptor antagonists
orphan	narcotic antagonists/agonists (m<u>orphinan</u> derivatives)
pred	<u>pred</u>nisone and <u>pred</u>nisolone derivatives
terol	bronchodilators (phenethylamine derivatives)
trop(ium)	<u>atrop</u>ine derivative (quaternary ammon<u>ium</u> salt)

Chapter 4: Immune

amivir	neuraminidase inhibitors
bendazole	anthelmintics (ti<u>bendazole</u> type)
cavir	carbocyclic nucleosides
cef	cephalosporins
cillin	peni<u>cillins</u>
citabine	nucleoside antiviral / antineoplastic agents, cytarabine or azarabine derivatives
conazole	systemic antifungals (mi<u>conazole</u> type)
cycline	antibiotics (tetra<u>cycline</u> derivatives)
cyclovir	antivirals (a<u>cyclovir</u> type)
floxacin	fluoroquinolone (not on Stem List)
kacin	antibiotics obtained from *Streptomyces kanamyceticus* (related to <u>kanamycin</u>)
lizumab	monoclonal antibodies
micin	antibiotics (*Micromonospora* strains)
mycin	antibiotics (*Streptomyces* strain)
navir	HIV protease inhibitors (saqui<u>navir</u> type)
nidazole	antiprotozoal substances (metro<u>nidazole</u> type)
nifur	5-<u>nitrofuran</u> derivatives
oxacin	antibacterials (quinolone derivatives)
oxanide	antiparasitics (salicylanilide derivatives)
prim	antibacterials (trimetho<u>prim</u> type)

rifa	antibiotics (<u>rifa</u>mycin derivatives)
sulfa	antimicrobials (<u>sulfona</u>mides derivatives)
tegravir	in<u>tegra</u>se inhibitors
thromycin	macrolide (not on Stem List)
vir	anti<u>vir</u>als
virenz	non-nucleoside reverse transcriptase inhibitors; benzoxazinone derivatives
viroc	CC chemokine receptor type 5 (CCR5) antagonists
vudine	antineoplastics; antivirals (zido<u>vudine</u> group) (exception: edoxudine)
zolid	oxa<u>zolid</u>inone antibacterials

Chapter 5: Neuro

azepam	antianxiety agents (di<u>azepam</u> type)
azolam	(WHO stem) diazepam derivatives
caine	local anesthetics
clone	hypnotics/tranquilizers (zopi<u>clone</u> type)
dopa	<u>dopa</u>mine receptor agonists
faxine	antianxiety, antidepressant inhibitor of norepinephrine and dopamine re-uptake
gab	<u>gab</u>amimetics
giline	Monoamine oxidase (MAO) inhibitors, type B
melteon	selective melatonin receptor agonist
oxetine	antidepressants (flu<u>oxetine</u> type)
peridol	antipsychotics (halo<u>peridol</u> type)
peridone	antipsychotics (ris<u>peridone</u> type)
pezil	acetylcholinesterase inhibitors used in the treatment of Alzheimer's disease
pidem	hypnotics/sedatives (zol<u>pidem</u> type)
pin(e)	tricyclic compounds
tiapine	antipsychotics (dibenzothiazepine derivatives)
toin	antiepileptics (hydan<u>toin</u> derivatives)
traline	selective serotonin reuptake inhibitors (SSRI)
triptyline	antidepressants (dibenzol[a,d] cycloheptane derivatives)
nicline	<u>ni</u>cotinic acetylcho<u>line</u> receptor partial agonists/agonists

barb	barbituric acid derivatives
spirone	anxiolytics (buspirone type)
fetamine	amfetamine derivatives
piprazole	(WHO stem) psychotropics, phenylpiperazine derivatives (future use is discouraged due to conflict with stem -prazole)
racetam	nootropic agents (learning, cognitive enhancers), piracetam type
sidone	antipsychotic with binding activity on serotonin (5-HT2A) and dopamine (D2) receptors
tropine	atropine derivatives; Subgroups: tertiary amines (e.g., benztropine)
mantine	antivirals/antiparkinsonians (adamantane derivatives)

Chapter 6: Cardio

alol	combined alpha and beta blockers
azosin	antihypertensives (prazosin type)
dil	vasodilators (undefined group)
dipine	phenylpyridine vasodilators (nifedipine type)
dralazine	antihypertensives (hydrazine-phthalazines)
farin	warfarin analogs
fibrate	antihyperlipidemics (clofibrate type)
gatran	thrombin inhibitors (argatroban type)
grel	platelet aggregation inhibitors, primarily platelet P2Y12 receptor antagonists
imibe	antihyperlipidaemics, acyl CoA: cholesterol acyltransferase (ACAT) inhibitors
iodarone	indicates high iodine content antiarrhythmic
nitro	(WHO stem) NO_2 derivatives
olol	beta-blockers (propranolol type)
pamil	coronary vasodilators (verapamil type)
parin	heparin derivatives and low molecular weight (or depolymerized) heparins
pril	antihypertensives (ACE inhibitors)
sartan	angiotensin II receptor antagonists
semide	diuretics (furosemide type)
thiazide	diuretics (thiazide derivatives)

tiazem	calcium channel blockers (dil<u>tiazem</u> type)
tril	endopeptidase inhibitors (e.g. neprilysin)
trop(ine)	atropine derivatives; Subgroups: tertiary amines (e.g., benz<u>tropine</u>)
vastatin	antihyperlipidemics (HMG-CoA inhibitors)
xaban	antithrombotics, blood coagulation factor XA inhibitors

Chapter 7: Endocrine / Misc.

afil	phosphodiesterase type 5 (PDE5) inhibitors
estr	<u>estr</u>ogens
fenacin	muscarinic receptor antagonists
formin	hypoglycemics (phen<u>formin</u> type)
gest	pro<u>gest</u>ins
gli (was gly)	antihyperglycemics
glinide	antidiabetic, sodium glucose co-transporter 2 (SGLT2) inhibitors, not phlorozin derivatives
gliptin	dipeptidyl aminopeptidase-IV inhibitors
glitazone	peroxisome proliferator activating receptor (PPAR) agonists (thiazolidene derivatives)
glutide	<u>gl</u>ucagon-like pep<u>tide</u> (GLP) analogs
gly	antihyper<u>gly</u>cemics
ster	<u>ster</u>oids (androgens, anabolics)
steride	testosterone reductase inhibitors
tide	pep<u>tide</u>s
uracil	<u>uracil</u> derivatives used as thyroid antagonists and as antineoplastics

GENERIC AND BRAND NAME INDEX

Generic and Brand Name Index

Manufactured by Amazon.ca
Acheson, AB

12820416R00337